Praise for McMoyler Method and *The Best Birth*

"McMoyler Method is unique and magical. My patients who have attended their classes are well prepared for all eventualities and uniformly joyous over their birth experience. The partners are comfortable in the delivery suite and fully engaged too."

—Laurie Green, MD,
Founding partner of the Pacific Women's Obstetrics and Gynecology Medical Group

"Pierre and I worked with Sarah before the birth of our first child, and her lessons have continued to benefit us through all of our pregnancies and births. McMoyler Method prepared us for labor and delivery, reduced our anxieties, and strengthened our connection to each other during the birth. We recommend her approach to anyone who wants to be more engaged and prepared for the wonderful journey of childbirth."

—Pam and Pierre Omidyar,
Founder of eBay

"When the time came to have our baby, my wife and I had to make a lot of decisions under pressure. Sarah's help was invaluable; she had us simulate different scenarios before the birth which helped potentially confusing and overwhelming situations seem familiar. The techniques in her program reminded me of the ways my Olympic coaches used to prepare us for the big event."

—Jonny Moseley,
Olympic Gold Medalist

"Sarah McMoyler leads the industry in her ability to bring the basics back to birthing with a welcomed combination of accessible practicality and judgment-free advice about today's options. I applaud her refreshingly modern commitment to the ultimate goal—healthy mom, healthy baby."

—Ali Wing,
Founder and CEO, www.giggle.com

"Our first McMoyler Method class was packed with information. We learned useful techniques to get me through the stages of labor, and my husband learned nearly how painful labor could be. We shared our stories, hopes, and fears and left feeling more confident about the birth process. McMoyler Method was so useful that when I was pregnant with our second child, we flew from Chicago to San Francisco just to repeat the course. It was more than a day's journey, but it was worth it!"

—Barb Brabec and Geoff Hansen,
Hollywood Assistant Director

"The greatest gift new parents can offer each other and their child is being emotionally and mentally aware, prepared, and present for the magic of delivery. Offering a realistic picture of every scenario expectant parents may face, McMoyler Method provides thoughtful, detailed alternatives and solutions that empower both parents to have the best birth possible."

—Alexis Swanson Traina,
Swanson Vineyards, proud mother of Johnny

"We were thoroughly enlightened and entertained by Sarah McMoyler's intensive course and the McMoyler Method. For many years the thought of labor was a bit frightening to us, but the techniques we learned and confidence that was built that day prepared us for our dream birth. Sarah is a true professional with an intense passion to empower and educate couples through the most amazing experience of their lives!"

—Christy and Jeff Campitelli,
Drummer for guitarist Joe Satriani

"Offering real-life techniques for labor and delivery, *The Best Birth* is God's gift to pregnant couples. Sarah McMoyler is a top-notch professional with an amazing talent for educating people. I used McMoyler Method in my deliveries—and it worked like magic. Every couple preparing for childbirth should get this book."

—Sharone Melamed,
Entertainment and Media Entrepreneur

THE BEST BIRTH

ALSO BY ARMIN BROTT

The Expectant Father: Facts, Tips, and Advice for Dads-to-Be

The New Father: A Dad's Guide to the First Year

Fathering Your Toddler: A Dad's Guide to the Second and Third Years

Fathering Your School-Age Child: A Dad's Guide to the Wonder Years, 3 to 9

Father for Life: A Journey of Joy, Challenge, and Change

The Single Father: A Dad's Guide to Parenting without a Partner

Throwaway Dads: The Myths and Barriers that Keep Men from Being the Fathers They Want to Be

Toolbox for New Dads (DVD)

THE BEST BIRTH

Your Guide to the Safest, Healthiest, Most Satisfying Labor and Delivery

Sarah McMoyler, RN, BSN
with Armin Brott

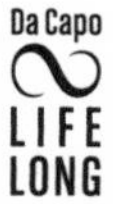

A Member of the Perseus Books Group

Many of the designations used by manufacturers and sellers to distinguish their products are claimed as trademarks. Where those designations appear in this book and Da Capo Press was aware of a trademark claim, the designations have been printed in initial capital letters.

Printed in the United States of America.

Designed by Brent Wilcox
Set in 11.25 point ITC New Baskerville by the Perseus Books Group

Library of Congress Cataloging-in-Publication Data
McMoyler, Sarah.
The best birth : your guide to the safest, healthiest, most satisfying labor and delivery / Sarah McMoyler with Armin Brott.
p. cm.
Includes bibliographical references and index.
ISBN-13: 978-0-7382-1121-3 (alk. paper)
1. Childbirth—Popular works. I. Brott, Armin A. II. Title.
RG525.M395 2008
618.2—dc22

2007050559

Published by Da Capo Press
A Member of the Perseus Books Group
www.dacapopress.com

Note: The information in this book is true and complete to the best of our knowledge. This book is intended only as an informative guide for those wishing to know more about health issues. In no way is this book intended to replace, countermand, or conflict with the advice given to you by your own health care provider. The ultimate decision concerning care should be made between you and your doctor. We strongly recommend you follow his or her advice. Information in this book is general and is offered with no guarantees on the part of the authors or Da Capo Press. The authors and publisher disclaim all liability in connection with the use of this book.

1 2 3 4 5 6 7 8 9

For my hearts, Jeff, Luke, and Corey
—SM

To Liz
—AB

Contents

CHAPTER

1

It's *Not* Your Mother's Birth Experience Anymore

FIRST AND FOREMOST, *congratulations!* However this happened—whether the stork landed unexpectedly on your rooftop, you planned your pregnancy, or you needed a little high-tech help along the way—you are embarking on what we consider to be the biggest event of your lives. Never mind the vacation, the wedding, the honeymoon, the new job, the new house, the new car. Nothing even comes close. Having a baby changes everything. Forever, and in more ways than you can imagine. From the joyful and heartwarming to the challenging and mind-bending, and everything in between.

Raising a child is a full-time job. As new parents, you and your partner will need to prepare for the unexpected, remain flexible, and work together as a team. It's no coincidence that that's also exactly what the two of you will need to do to get through labor and delivery. You may be looking into some of the traditional childbirth prep classes and methods to help you navigate these unfamiliar waters. Unfortunately, traditional childbirth courses won't give you the knowledge, training, or preparation you need.

Introducing McMoyler Method

For more than fifty years, the childbirth education field has been dominated by two methods: Lamaze and Bradley. Although there's no question that both were revolutionary in their time, today they're hopelessly out of date, still preparing couples to give birth using last century's approaches, attitudes, and assumptions. Unmedicated childbirth is often seen as the only "normal" way to have a baby, and the new mother is left feeling guilty and/or inadequate unless she delivers without drugs or interventions of any kind. At the end of the day, that attitude undermines what should be the most wonderful and powerful memories of a couple's lifetime.

Well, move over, Lamaze and Bradley, there's a new childbirth method in town.

Welcome to McMoyler Method, *the* childbirth method for the twenty-first century. McMoyler Method teaches today's busy expectant couples exactly what they need to know to have a positive birth experience and jumpstart their new life as a family.

McMoyler Method is *not* a collection of techniques for managing birth, and it doesn't provide a specific checklist of things students must do during labor and delivery or risk failing. Instead, McMoyler Method is a powerful *philosophy,* one that will act as the foundation for teaching you and your partner the must-know details about the birth process, giving you the knowledge and tools you need to make the right decisions for yourselves and your baby every step of the way.

Mental and emotional preparation are paramount, because no one can predict exactly what's going to happen on the day you give birth. Not your doctor, not your mother, not your sister, or your neighbor, or even those annoying strangers who think it's okay to fondle your pregnant belly. Only the stork knows for sure.

McMoyler Method explodes the myths of childbirth prep as we know it, myths that have been passed down to millions of couples who have ended up with less-than-satisfying childbirth experiences, feeling disappointed and regretful. *In McMoyler Method, there's no such thing as a less-than-satisfying experience. The only objective is "healthy mom, healthy baby—however you get there."*

Here are the basic tenets of McMoyler Method:

- You will be able to trust the health care team to guide you through your entire birth experience.
- You may want a "natural" childbirth, avoiding interventions, and McMoyler Method supports that. We believe your body is built to give birth and that it deserves every opportunity to do so without intervention.
- You have access to viable pain-management options.
- You may need to utilize medical advancements to ensure a healthy delivery.
- Your partner is essential to the delivery process.
- You both will be transformed, regardless of how your baby is born.
- You will cherish the memory of this day for the rest of your lives.
- Childbirth preparation should be scientifically sound and reality-based, providing a thorough knowledge of current medical options and approaches.
- Classes should be taught by a licensed medical professional. If not, you risk getting little more than theory, personal opinion, and speculation. Most Lamaze and Bradley instructors are laypeople with limited medical training, who may have attended a few dozen births. On the other hand, a trained labor and delivery nurse has attended hundreds if not thousands.

You're Not in This Alone

At the very core of the McMoyler Method philosophy is the idea that the dad-to-be belongs front and center. He's no longer a nice-to-have observer, limited to holding hands, bringing ice chips, directing breathing patterns, or hiding behind the camera. He's a must-have participant with an essential role to play. (It's important to note here that in this regard, McMoyler Method owes a debt of gratitude to Lamaze and Bradley, who turned the childbirth industry on its head by taking dads out of the waiting room and encouraging them to participate. However, what was so revolutionary just a few decades ago doesn't go nearly far enough today.)

With McMoyler Method, your partner will learn that childbirth is not a spectator sport. (It could, however, be considered an extreme sport.) It's going to be the toughest, longest day of your life, and you will want and need him for unconditional support and guidance and to help make decisions along the way. By reading this book (or at least the sections that are written specifically for him), he'll learn all the twists and turns labor can take, and the exciting and exhausting facts.

He'll learn about everything that could possibly happen during labor and delivery. He'll learn exactly what to do with you during contractions, as well as the critical spaces between them, when you're literally catching your breath. He'll understand how to work with the health care team; how to make informed and responsible decisions; and how to be present, involved, and encouraging throughout. He'll also learn practical strategies and tips to help you keep labor moving forward.

McMoyler Method focuses so much attention on the partners, because, frankly, they aren't going to be having uterine contractions. Labor is a physical, emotional, sometimes spiritual experience, and you won't have the wherewithal in the middle of it to go through the file drawers of your brain trying to remember what we've told you about coping with active labor contractions. Partners, on the other hand, will be able to help guide you, reassure you, and work with the health care professionals to make sure that you have everything you need along the way.

A NOTE ABOUT PARTNERS

At our flagship location in San Francisco, it has been our privilege to prepare over 10,000 people to give birth. These couples have come in all shapes and sizes, colors and configurations. What they all have in common, though, is that one person was pregnant and the other was in a supporting role. Although the majority of those support people have been husbands, many have not (we've had mothers, sisters, good friends, doulas, boyfriends, fiancés, lovers, and more). From our perspective, it doesn't matter who that person is, just as long as he or she will be there to provide the mom-to-be with unconditional support and guidance. That said, we've opted to refer to that support person as "husband" or "partner."

To get a better idea of the difference between a McMoyler Method couple and one that has been through one of the standard childbirth prep courses, consider this: Having a great birth experience is like having the wedding of your dreams. (I know that some readers aren't married, and this analogy isn't meant as a judgment. Even if you've been only a *guest* at a wedding, I think you'll understand where I'm going with this.) Here's how:

- You've probably had a vision in your mind, maybe for years, of how you want the big event to go.

- When you finally meet the man of your dreams, the two of you begin preparing for this momentous occasion.
- You talk together endlessly, comparing and contrasting each other's ideas.
- You talk with friends and family about their weddings.
- You scout locations, and you hire professionals to handle all the details, including performing the ceremony.
- You have a plan B, just in case something doesn't happen like you thought it would.
- If your beautifully planned outdoor ceremony gets rained out, or something else happens and you have to implement plan B (or C or D), you go through with it anyway.
- When you think back to all the stress and tension and anxiety that went into the planning, you have to laugh. Sure, when all is said and done, there were a few hitches, but at the end of the day, everything was perfect: the moment, the day, the man, the memory . . .

As I said at the very beginning of this chapter, we believe that having a baby is the biggest event of your lives, bar none. And that's why I encourage you and your partner to spend at least as much time—if not more—preparing yourselves (and each other) for it.

Who's Behind McMoyler Method, Anyway?

Although McMoyler Method got its official start in 1994, the seeds that produced it were planted many years before, when my husband, Jeff, and I arrived at the hospital to give birth to our first child. Even though I was a labor and delivery nurse myself, and Jeff and I had taken the requisite classes to prepare for the birth, it wasn't until we were well into the labor that we realized that what we'd been taught had very little to do with what was actually happening. My husband was very uncomfortable during the many hours of labor and the multitude of medical procedures.

After one of many pelvic exams and many hours of labor, I was told that I was still only 3 centimeters dilated. I said, "Enough! Get the anesthesiologist, and get him *now.*" Thanks to the epidural, I got some much-needed rest, and when it came time to push that baby out, I was feeling energized and ready to go.

Even though I had seen hundreds of babies born, nothing compared to the experience of giving birth. It's as amazing as people say it is—all the hours of sweat and tears in labor truly seemed to vanish. I will never, ever forget that day (or the day his brother was born two years later).

When I came back to work after my maternity leave, I found that my bedside nursing care was dramatically changed. What I recalled from my own experience was that Jeff was nowhere near prepared enough to have been actively involved in labor and delivery. I know for a fact that he wished he would have been able to participate more. It wasn't that he didn't want to be part of the process or support and help me, it was just that he had no idea how to do it. No one had shown him how to get started.

As a labor and delivery nurse, I had seen the same scene unfold day in and day out at work. Patient after patient would roll through the doors. The women—most of whom had been through traditional childbirth prep classes—were clueless about how to cope with contractions. The partners (most of whom were at the very same classes) had no idea how to help and guide the expectant mother. And neither of them knew how to evaluate their options, make decisions along the way, or effectively work with the health care team. Clearly there was something missing—for me, my husband, and millions of other couples. The traditional ways of preparing couples for childbirth simply weren't working. There was far too much fear, confusion, and dissatisfaction.

I now found myself approaching my patients in labor very differently: getting husbands out of their chairs over by the window and summoning them to the bedside, inviting them to lend support, showing them what to do, including them in what was going on. I needed their help, and moms-to-be wanted them nearby.

I realized that what today's couples really need is a new approach, one that teaches them everything they need to know (as opposed to what's just nice to know) about labor and delivery, and truly prepares them for the biggest event of their lives. Although I could continue reaching one couple at a time, I wanted to take this message to a far bigger audience. So I hung out my own shingle and began teaching what would eventually be called McMoyler Method.

How Is *The Best Birth* Different from a McMoyler Method Class?

This book is *not* designed to be a McMoyler Method course in a box. You won't have a chance to see your partner on his hands and knees, playing the part of a woman in labor. You won't be able to watch the video footage of actual labors and births. What you *will* get is the benefit of my twenty-plus years as a labor and delivery nurse and childbirth educator. And, more important, because McMoyler Method courses and *The Best Birth* share the same philosophy, you'll finish reading armed with the same knowledge and must-know information that in-class students receive.

Does McMoyler Method Have an Agenda?

No. McMoyler Method strongly supports low- to no-intervention births—as long as that's what's best for everyone—and in giving your body a fair chance to do the work it was built to do. On the other hand, if your mind and body are fatigued beyond belief and labor isn't progressing, it's time to consider other options.

With most traditional childbirth methods (including Bradley and Lamaze), women are expected to have a "natural" or "normal," unmedicated childbirth. Opting for an epidural or any other pain medication is considered a failure. And having a cesarean requires a "grieving period" (as Lamaze suggests) to mourn the loss of the perfect birth. Personally, I think that making new parents feel guilty if they don't live up to some pie-in-the-sky fantasy birth scenario is an absolutely unnecessary way to get them started on the biggest adventure of their lives. That's why with McMoyler Method, there's no such thing as failure. If a cesarean is the safest choice, we're thankful that the option exists and see it as a cause for relief, not grief.

McMoyler Method advocates reality-based preparation. *No guilt, no failure, no politics, no agenda—know your options.* Sometimes just knowing there's a safety net in place can make it easier to make it through. It's absolutely fine to see yourself working through labor on your own steam, although we strongly recommend being reminded along the way that you have options available to you. The safety net comes in many forms; just remember that it's there if you need it.

Sadly, the "natural or nothing" attitude refuses to die. And as a result, instead of enjoying their new role as parents, millions of couples are overwhelmed with feelings of disappointment and regret.

What You'll Learn in This Book

Let me give you a quick overview of what you (and your partner) will learn over the course of the rest of *The Best Birth*:

In Chapter 2 we'll dive right into the number-one concern expectant mothers have: pain, specifically, how much and for how long. (After all, she's going into the hospital to do something that's guaranteed to be painful and she has no idea how long it'll last. Who *wouldn't* be concerned?) We'll talk about the critical role fear plays in increasing pain. We'll discuss medical and nonmedical pain-management options, and we'll learn what works and what doesn't (hint: breathing patterns that are taught in traditional childbirth prep classes don't). Finally, you'll learn more than a dozen techniques that can help you better cope with your pain and keep labor progressing.

Chapter 3 is devoted to Dad, partner, support person, whoever that individual will be—what his role is and why he's so essential to the process. We'll begin by comparing a dad who has been through a traditional childbirth prep course to a McMoyler Method dad. We'll talk about how his involvement sets the stage for becoming a family, including tips for getting even the most reluctant dad involved. In this chapter I'll introduce the concept of doulas and why I suggest that you *don't* hire one (hint: Dad is a better companion).

Hand this book over to your partner and have him read Chapter 4, which will give him the specifics on how to stay involved from now until the baby is born. He'll learn (perhaps more than he bargained for) about the various bodily functions that he'll be exposed to during labor and delivery, and nine McMoyler Maneuvers—techniques he'll be able to use to help you cope and to help labor progress.

The next two chapters focus on the medical team. In Chapter 5 you'll learn that the medical team is *not* the enemy, that they have the very same goals you do: healthy moms and healthy babies. In this chapter, we'll expose the truth behind some of the little, not-so-white lies of childbirth, such as: *Having a baby at home provides a more satisfying birth experience.* Maybe. Unless something unexpected and unanticipated occurs, which sometimes does at the very end. Often by that time, you may be too far from the hospital to get the help you need. *Epidurals lead to cesareans.* Most likely not. Loooong labors lead to cesareans. *Doctors do episiotomies for their own convenience.* Not true. If the doctor can deliver over an intact perineum (or with a small tear), he or she will be congratulating you and out the door sooner than if he or she had cut an episiotomy. *Doctors push cesareans for their own convenience.* In fact, it is highly *in*convenient to do a cesarean; furthermore, hospitals tend to lose money on a surgical delivery. Many hospitals across the country have quality-assurance committees responsible for reviewing every cesarean. They want to know: what was the diagnosis and what was the outcome.

In Chapter 6 you'll meet every person on the medical team and learn what they do and why. You'll learn the lingo of labor and delivery: Apgar? Cephalopelvic disproportion? Effacement? Fetal distress? Station? Oxytocin? Perineum? Ruptured membranes? You'll get a clear definition of these and several dozen more common terms you're likely to hear in the hours before your baby is born. The more you know, the more involved you can be in the process. We'll talk about the most common interventions—including the big three: induction, epidural, and cesarean—what they are, why they happen, and what the advantages and disadvantages are. We'll end the chapter with some specific strategies you can use to quickly develop close working relationships with the entire hospital medical team. You have no idea how amazingly helpful they can be.

When you arrive at the hospital to deliver your baby, there is absolutely no way to predict exactly how your labor will progress or the birth will take place. In Chapter 7 we'll talk about the importance of keeping your expectations reasonable and focusing on the result (a baby) instead of how you get to the finish line (whether you have a natural/unmedicated birth, epidural, or a cesarean). We'll talk quite a bit about birth plans and how walking into the hospital with a rigid birth plan can create some unintended tension with the medical team. A birth plan can also set you up for feeling that you've failed if you don't follow it to the letter. As we've said before, with McMoyler Method, there's no such thing as failure. The best plan is to learn as much as you can in advance so that throughout the birth process, you can both work with your health care team to make the decisions that are right for *you*.

Over the course of many years spent in labor and delivery and the hundreds of hours teaching expectant couples, I've found that women have a deep curiosity about other women's birth experiences. So in Chapter 8 you'll hear the unvarnished stories of women who've been there. Some had the picture-perfect birth. For others, almost *nothing* went according to plan. What all these stories have in common is that the new parents kept their eyes on the prize and left the hospital with memories for a lifetime.

Throughout the book, you will find key points to focus on, including:

- **DadBoxes,** which contain tips written specifically for dad/partner that will help him better understand what's going on, how he can be involved, and exactly what to be doing.

- **Prenatal prep work:** homework assignments you'll actually want to do. Does anyone who takes a traditional childbirth class actually go home and practice breathing patterns? I doubt it. So instead, I suggest that you and your partner have an ongoing series of discussions. To make this a little easier, I've included conversation starters that will get you talking about critical issues, such as: what your biggest concerns are; what *you* need to get you through this process; what your thoughts are about epidurals, cesareans, and other interventions; and how you envision your partner being involved.

To sum it up, every chapter in *The Best Birth* will reduce your stress and anxiety, and provide you and your husband with the specific tools and the knowledge you'll need to achieve the healthiest, safest, most satisfying labor and delivery.

CHAPTER 2

Yes, Virginia, It's Going to Hurt

WHAT YOU'LL LEARN IN THIS CHAPTER:

- Pain: how much and for how long
- The connection between fear and pain
- What actually causes pain, and how to cope with it
- Pain-management options that really work
- How your partner and the healthcare team will help you make the decisions that are best for *you*

AT THE BEGINNING of every Childbirth 101 class, we always ask people to tell us what concerns them most about labor and delivery. The answers are almost always the same. Moms say they're afraid that, one, they'll lose control, and two, it'll hurt like hell. Dads worry that they won't be able to help the woman they love cope with the pain. The moms are right on both counts. The dads couldn't be more wrong.

Breaking the Cycle

The most important thing to know about pain is that it's the first step in a nasty cycle that can bring labor to a grinding halt and set the stage for panic. This cycle—fear, tension, pain—was first proposed by British obstetrician Grantley Dick-Read in his 1932 book, *Childbirth without Fear.*

Here's how it works: When you feel afraid, your body gives you a jolt of adrenaline and goes into "fight or flight" mode, diverting as much blood as it can to your arms and legs so you can get away from whatever it is that's making you afraid (that's why people who are frightened are often "white as a sheet"). All the extra blood that just went to your arms and legs really belongs in the muscles that make up your uterus and create contractions. The result is a blood-starved uterus that can't do its job. That slows labor and at the same time causes pain.

Fortunately, nature provides a break between contractions that is designed to give you a chance to release the built-up tension and regain some of your strength. Labor pain is unique in that it goes on for so long and often does not progress efficiently; this is when women can spiral into a vicious cycle: Your fear of the next contraction will make you tense up. That releases even more adrenaline, which tightens your muscles and increases the pain even more. That makes it next to impossible for you to rest during the downtimes. And without the recovery time between contractions, you'll have even more anticipatory tension, creating more fear, more tension, more pain . . . and so it goes.

For most first-time moms, labor is like running a marathon. It takes a lot of time and a lot of endurance. Without constant reminders about how to cope with contractions, without using the brief respites along the way, chances are you'll run out of steam and quickly reach your mental and physical limits. When that happens, you'll run into a brick wall. And from there, it's only a hop, skip, and a jump to panic and hysteria, as you anxiously wonder how the @#$%! you'll *ever* get through this.

> *At one point, I was dilated 8 centimeters. I was exhausted and starting to come undone. My husband got in my face and in between contractions kept repeating, "You can do this," "You are doing it," "The baby is coming." I remember the nurse kneeling beside him and together they helped me get through the mind-bending peaks of the contractions and then to completely relax in between. It was the hardest thing I've ever done. If the labor had not moved along and I'd gotten stuck at any point, I would have definitely considered an epidural.*
>
> —RACHEL K., NEW MOM

The fear-tension-pain cycle is a chicken-and-egg kind of thing, and it doesn't really matter which one came first. Imagine that you're standing on the edge of a cliff. Any step, whether it's fear or tension or pain, could push you over. And once you start falling, it's very hard to stop. Fortunately, there are effective ways of coping with the pain that will reduce the fear and tension and help you take a few steps away from the precipice. I'll tell you exactly how later in this chapter, but first let's talk a little bit about some of the pain relief/management/coping strategies that *don't* work.

Pain Relief Myths

Traditional childbirth methods have adopted two almost contradictory philosophies about pain. First, that breathing techniques take away the pain. Second, that pain is a good thing and it helps labor progress. It's time to debunk both of these myths.

Breathing

There's no question that breathing is important. On the most basic level, when you inhale, oxygen is absorbed through the lungs into your blood and goes out to nourish every cell in your body. Oxygen-starved muscles, the uterus included, don't perform well and lead to fatigue and a perception of increased pain.

Yoga practitioners and people who meditate have understood for centuries the great long-term and short-term benefits of controlled, slow, deep breathing. Studies have shown that in the long run, regular deep breathing can reduce blood pressure and hypertension and help manage stress. In the short run, the same kind of breathing can calm and center you, help you get through moments of tension and anxiety, and increase your ability to cope with pain.

But what breathing *can't* do is *remove* the kind of pain you're likely to have with every contraction. Traditional childbirth methods maintain that special breathing patterns can help overcome (or at least minimize) labor pain. And so they tell expectant couples to practice fast-paced "he-he-he," "whoo-whoo-whoo," or any number of other combinations of monosyllabic words. In my experience, this simply does not work to affect pain or increase your ability to cope.

> *When my wife was pregnant with our first child, we took a childbirth prep class through the hospital. We learned a ton about labor and delivery and came home with a bunch of breathing patterns I was supposed to help my wife with during contractions. When we got to the hospital, things didn't go quite as planned. The breathing stuff didn't work at all and she started to panic. Things just escalated from there, and we ended with exactly what we didn't want: a cesarean. We weren't sure who to turn to for help, and I had no idea what to do. We thought we were prepared, but boy, were we wrong.*
>
> —ERIC B., NEW DAD

As mentioned above, for breathing to do anything at all to reduce stress or anxiety or tension or pain, the breaths have to be controlled, slow, and deep. "He-he-he" and "whoo-whoo-whoo" are shallow, and shallow breathing doesn't get the oxygen where it needs to go. The result is more tension and anxiety. And those lead to, yep, pain. A little later in this chapter, we'll talk about the McMoyler Method alternative—which really can enhance coping.

Pain Is Good—Not!

In recent years, Lamaze and Bradley have begun to distance themselves from breathing patterns as a pain coping mechanism. In my view, that's a good thing. But I strongly object to some of the other changes they've made. For example, a recent article on pregnancy-info.net made this startling claim: "Contrary to what many people may believe, Lamaze does not actually aim to make the labor process less painful. In fact, the Lamaze philosophy believes that the pain you experience during labor acts as a protective force for your body." (I wonder what Dr. Lamaze himself, whose book, *Painless Childbirth,* was the basis of the Lamaze method, would say about that.) The Lamaze Web site (lamaze.org) reiterates that point and goes even further: "Some women find that experiencing and coping with the pain of labor and birth is similar to the hard work demanded by dancers and athletes. Lamaze classes help women understand the value of pain and learn how to respond to pain in ways that both facilitate labor and increase comfort."

As someone who has both had children and run marathons, I agree that the two are somewhat similar in terms of the amount of strength and endurance required, and the feeling of triumph that comes at the finish line. And I can go along with "facilitate labor."

As far as "increase comfort" goes, I'd change the word to "coping," since there's nothing comfortable about labor. I often have to explain the difference to expectant dads who mistakenly think their job is to make their wife more comfortable during labor. That just is not going to happen. What he can do, though, is help her cope, one contraction at a time.

I even understand the notion that pain in some contexts has value. If you pull a muscle or have a stomachache, your body uses pain to tell you that you need to *stop* doing something. What is labor pain trying to tell you, besides that you should stop being pregnant?

> *I had my baby naturally and it was the most physically demanding thing I've ever done. I felt incredibly proud of myself at having done it on my own. I really think now that having been through that experience, there's nothing I can't do.*
>
> —HELEN V., NEW MOM

Yes, pain in childbirth is natural. But despite some people's attempts to romanticize it or make it "satisfying" or "a gift," or their suggestions that giving birth without medical pain relief will make you a better person or a "real woman," pain is most certainly *not* necessary. And it's also not the foundation on which you'll build the memory of a lifetime (which we'll discuss in Chapter 7).

WHAT, EXACTLY, CAUSES PAIN DURING LABOR?

There are two kinds of pain during labor: physical and psychological/emotional. Here's what's going on physiologically that actually causes pain.

- Effacement and dilation of the cervix
- Pressure of the baby's head as it descends through the birth canal and pelvis

- Lactic acid buildup as the uterus contracts
- Pressure from the contracting uterus on the bladder, rectum, fallopian tubes, ovaries, and ligaments
- Size and position of the baby
- Stretching of the vagina and perineum

Okay, It Hurts, But What Does That Mean?

New mothers usually put childbirth at the top of their list of most painful experiences. Keep in mind that pain is a very subjective thing, and what one woman may describe as "mild" or "tolerable," another may say was "horrible" or "mind-numbing." Labor pain is also different from a lot of other kinds of pain. (At the very least, when it's over, you get a great reward: your baby. After most other kinds of pain, all you get is a scar.) What makes it especially difficult is not so much the intensity of the pain itself, but rather that it goes on for so long. And instead of fading with time, the contractions get more painful and last longer. That said, there are a number of factors that we know can influence your *perception* of the severity of your pain and how long it lasts.

- **Expectations.** We're bombarded with images about how painful childbirth is. Just think of the "births" you've seen on television in sitcoms or dramas. The pain is usually shown as excruciating, but it only lasts until the next commercial. The clips you may have seen in a childbirth prep class leave a longer-lasting impression because you know what you're seeing is real. And then there are the books pregnant women read, some of which you may have on your shelf right now. According to Marci Lobel, Ph.D., director of the Stony Brook Pregnancy Project at Stony Brook University, "Popular books written for pregnant women often understate the degree of pain experienced during birth, and may overstate the effectiveness of childbirth preparation in reducing pain." When pre-labor expectations are close to during-labor reality, women tend to rate their pain as less severe.

- **Whether you've taken a childbirth prep course.** Most women have never truly experienced pain (no, paper cuts don't count), and it's hard to prepare your body and mind for a guaranteed-painful situation if you have no frame of reference. Taking a class is no guarantee that you'll experience less pain. McMoyler Method is committed to presenting the full range of possibilities; be prepared for whatever the stork has in mind for you. Given the fact that labor is going to be painful, you will want to begin preparing, discussing, and setting realistic goals long before the day of delivery.
- **Fear and anxiety.** If your prenatal education hasn't actually prepared you for labor by teaching you a variety of pain-management options (which will *not* be the case by the time you're done with this book), the entire painful process will become frightening and you'll rate it as much more severe.
- **Confidence.** Confidence that your expectations are reasonable, that your partner will be there for you throughout, that he and the medical team will support and guide you and help you make the best decisions for you and the baby; confidence that if you need pain relief, you'll get it.
- **Support.** Having your partner or other trusted person there to support and encourage and praise you will make the whole experience more doable and will underscore the very important concept that you're doing this *together.* He will help you cope with the intense peak of each contraction and release and recuperate during the pain-free times in between.

- **Trust.** Having trust that your partner and the medical staff will get you through labor is an important base to be able to spring from. Continue asking questions prenatally of your partner and your OB/midwife until you feel secure in the fact that they are on your side and have you covered.
- **The baby's position.** The "ideal" position for the baby is head down, facing your back (referred to as anterior). In this position, the narrowest portion of the baby's head is descending first, where it fits better through your pelvis. The baby's soft, moldable face comes down against your backbone, so it's less intense for you. As the head descends, it puts necessary pressure on the opening cervix, helping it dilate, which means less time in labor. Having the baby facing your front ("sunny side up," or posterior position) produces what's called back labor. In that position, the largest part of the baby's head is trying to make its way through the pelvis, and the baby's bony skull is pressing, bone-against-bone, on your spine. That creates a double whammy: uterine contractions in the front, and painful back labor behind you. This combination is often the culprit in the very long labors that don't make steady progress. It's not impossible to deliver a posterior baby vaginally, but it's a pretty tall order. Some moms will end up with a cesarean for what I often refer to as WCO—won't come out.
- **How labor progresses.** That depends on the strength and regularity of the contractions, how well the cervix is dilating, and whether the baby is descending toward the birth canal. Labor that "fails to progress" tends to be more painful than steadily progressing labor, largely because it's going to seem like it goes on and on and on and on.

- **Your age.** There's no question that your body is built to give birth. However, there are some age-related differences. First-time moms generally report more pain than second-timers (in part, at least, because second labors are usually much shorter than the first). First-time mothers in their twenties generally have shorter labors than women in their thirties and forties, mostly because younger moms' bodies often labor more efficiently. With more and more women in their thirties and forties becoming pregnant, it is important to reinforce that many will give birth vaginally, specifically because high-tech help is there to assist the process. Granted, some of those moms will have a cesarean birth . . . at the end of the day, it was not the route they delivered their babies that mattered, but the result!
- **Your sensitivity to pain.** It's almost impossible to predict someone's pain tolerance, and often Mom's limited experience with any pain doesn't correlate to the pain of labor. One thing is certain: As labor moves forward and your contractions get longer and stronger, you will perceive them as more painful.

Pain Relief: What *Does* Work?

People have a tendency to think about pain relief as an either-or kind of thing: Either you have a completely unmedicated birth or you have an epidural the moment labor begins and eliminate the pain altogether. In McMoyler Method, you don't have to choose one or the other. Instead, we recommend making decisions along the way, depending on the degree of pain, how long the labor is going on, and how well you and the baby are tolerating it. Those factors, of course, will be different for every woman. It often comes down to one big question: time—"How long do I have to endure this?"

In this section, we're going to talk about nonmedical and medical approaches that will help you cope with your pain and keep the fear-tension-pain cycle from kicking in. If your goal is a completely "natural" birth, great, I'm all for it. If you think you might need an epidural, that's okay too. If you want something in between or to combine the two, that's fine. The most important thing is that you understand your options in advance and that you keep an open mind. Flexibility is key.

The worst time to try to make a pain-relief decision is at the peak of a contraction. Labor is a physical, emotional, and sometimes even spiritual experience. It is *not* cognitive, and you will *not* necessarily be pulling up what you read in this book. Your partner, on the other hand, will be thinking a bit more clearly. He will be able to work with the medical team to help you cope with your pain, making good decisions along the way, in response to your individual needs.

Nonmedical Options

Nonmedical coping strategies come in two basic categories: emotional and physical. I'm listing them briefly here; because most of them involve your partner, we'll discuss them in much greater detail in Chapter 4, Game Plans for Dads.

Emotional Coping Strategies

- **In-your-face mirroring.** When you're in active labor, you're going to be too preoccupied with simply getting through the contractions to listen to long explanations of what you should and shouldn't do to cope with the pain. As intensity builds, you will need clear and direct demonstration on how to get through the contraction. That's why we have your husband get nose-to-nose with you and actively demonstrate what it is that *you* need to do, whether it's making guttural moaning sounds during contractions or dropping your shoulders and unclenching your jaw in between. These techniques will make the peaks of the contractions more manageable and will help you utilize the break *between* contractions to recover and build up the energy you need to tackle the next one.

- **Engage the mind.** From the neck down, your body is built to give birth. The problem is with the brain, which tends to generate thoughts like "I don't want to do this," "I shouldn't be doing this," "I can't do this," "Someone make this stop," and "Get me out of here." Having something to focus on—your husband's face, a new environment or position—during contractions can really help.
- **Verbal anesthesia**. Between the length of time labor lasts and the intensity of the pain, it's easy to get bogged down in self-doubt. Between contractions, hearing words of encouragement, praise, excitement, support, and love from your husband goes a long way toward replenishing your rapidly depleting emotional and physical reserves.
- **Holding and reassuring**. (Technically, this is physical, but the effect is emotional.) This is particularly useful *in between* contractions, as most women don't really like being touched during contractions. If this is true for you, be sure to tell your husband.
- **Relinquish control.** Your body sets the pace of labor and the level of pain; the baby is coming out when she's good and ready. This is a big one for many women, especially those who are used to being in control of their life and everything

in it. Unfortunately, labor and delivery is pretty much out of your control. The more you can let go, trust your body to do what it's supposed to, and accept the support from your husband and the medical team, the sooner your baby will come out. Insisting on being in control or trying to micromanage labor tends to have the exact opposite effect, creating more frustrations and slowing it down even more.

DadBox

Hugging, stroking, massaging, and other kinds of touch are all excellent ways to be supportive and express love and compassion during labor. The trick is in the timing. Most women don't particularly like to be touched during a contraction—they're focusing on just getting through it, and too much touching can become annoying. Timing is everything. . . . There are two solutions. First, unless your wife specifically asks for it, keep your hands to yourself except during the all-important spaces between contractions. Second, spend some time now, long before labor starts, "practicing" hugs, massages, etc. Ask her what feels good, and what doesn't. Learn which parts of her body tend to be more tense than others, how much pressure she likes, and for how long. (Keep in mind that what worked well prenatally or in early labor may not work at all during active labor.)

One warning: In the midst of a contraction, your wife may say some things that could sting. A lot. Remember that she's going through the most intense experience of her life and is summoning up every ounce of strength and willpower to keep it together during those contractions. You're just going to have to take my word—your support means everything.

Physical Coping Strategies

- **Exercise**. Unless your doctor has said otherwise, you should exercise regularly while you're pregnant. At the very least it can strengthen your muscles and increase your stamina.

This is *not* the time to start a brand-new, intensive exercise regime, though. Continue doing what your body is used to, and pay close attention to how you're handling the exercise, particularly as the pregnancy progresses. I strongly recommend that you check with your OB/midwife to let her know what kind of exercise you're doing, how often, and for how long. Your body will let you know if it's no longer tolerating an activity. You might, for example, experience some uterine contractions, an elevated heart rate, or fatigue.

- **Music.** There is longstanding agreement that music provides a sense of soothing during labor. McMoyler Method recommends that long before labor strikes, you and your partner spend time listening to music you love and use it as a way to connect with each other. An added bonus to bringing music with you to the hospital is that when the health care team walks into your room and hears *your* music, they're now entering and becoming a part of your environment. This may sound like a small benefit, but it's actually quite remarkable in its ability to create continuity.
- **Aromatherapy**. Again, before labor starts you need to identify scents you love—and let your partner know. Usually subtle, mild scents provide an increased feeling of calm and reassurance during labor.
- **Massage.** As labor intensifies, massage (back, hands, feet, neck) is helpful between contractions. This is something you can certainly start doing now. It's important that you communicate to your husband what's working and what's not. If you don't tell him, there's no way he can do what works for you. Communication is especially important here because what hits the spot right now might be very different from what appeals to you in labor.

- **Hydration.** Most hospitals will provide juice, Popsicles, broth, Jell-O, tea, and water. You'll need to have some of each in between contractions, as the combination of fluids and sugar provides the energy you need for the long haul. You and the baby will fare far better when you're well hydrated. (Some women will need more fluids than they can actually drink and an IV may become necessary.)
- **Regular bathroom breaks.** Pressure on the bladder can inhibit progress and increase discomfort, so it's best to empty it at least once every hour. In early labor you'll be able to do this on your own. As the contractions intensify, your husband or nurse will need to help you get situated on the toilet. See page 84 in Chapter 4 for more on what we call the toilet trick.
- **Rest.** Get as much rest as possible in early labor and in between contractions as labor intensifies. If labor begins during the day, I suggest that you and your husband go out. Have one last meal together, go see a movie, or just take a walk. On the other hand, if labor begins in the middle of the night, try to doze off—or at least rest—in between contractions. Don't worry about trying to do anything to get labor to progress—labor has a mind of its own; the contractions will come.
- **Get up, walk, rock, change positions**. This is one of McMoyler Method's mantras. Being upright, out of the labor bed, and in motion is the best way to keep labor progressing. It helps dilate (open) and efface (thin) your cervix, and helps the baby descend into the birth canal. It also allows your pelvis to expand (it has been gradually expanding throughout the pregnancy, and over the entire course of labor, it can "give" as much as 25 percent more—and you want every bit of it). We've come up with nine specific up-and-about strategies that we call McMoyler Maneuvers. Trying a new one every forty-five

minutes or so will help you cope with the pain and keep labor moving forward. The McMoyler Maneuvers include the following; you'll find a complete list in Chapter 4:

1. The slow dance (you hang on your husband as if you were dancing at your high school prom)
2. Rocking chair and squatting (both help open the pelvis and allow the baby to descend)
3. Toilet trick (the hard toilet seat offers helpful counterpressure)
4. Shower power (uses the proven approach of hydrotherapy to cope during contractions and relax in between)

GO AHEAD, IMPROVISE

One of the funniest births I attended was with a woman who was moving along in labor, her partner willing to do whatever he could. She had spent a lot of time in the shower and made it to the pushing stage on her own steam, when all hell broke loose. She found pushing to be way more intense than coping with contractions, and was starting to freak out, and wanted an epidural right then. The anesthesiologist was in the operating room and unavailable.

So we got her positioned in the bed to begin pushing. She was giving it her all. Her husband was at the head of the bed, supporting her to curl in with each push, and I was positioned on the delivery stool at the foot of the bed, assessing how effective her pushes were.

All of a sudden, completely out of the blue, she burst into song, and at the top of her lungs she started belting out, "I've got that joy, joy, joy, joy, deep in my heart, deep in my heart, deep in my heart/I've got that joy, joy, joy, joy, deep in my heart, deep in my heart to stay!" Her husband started singing with her, and when she looked down the bed and locked eyes with me, I felt I had no choice but to sing along with them. It was like some odd scene out of a movie. (I glanced over at the pediatrician, who was standing by to assess the soon-to-be-born baby, and he said, "I don't sing.") The baby was born, with what felt like the Hallelujah chorus welcoming him into the world. True story, fond memory.

> *I used all of the McMoyler Maneuvers—sitting in the rocking chair and on the toilet, slow dancing with my husband, the birthing ball, and squatting. But the one that worked best for me was getting on my hands and knees—with my husband—in the warm shower. I tell you, it made all the difference, just to not be alone and have him sort of carry me through each one. I'm not sure it reduced the pain, but it certainly made it easier to deal with. . . . I couldn't have done it without him. Best of all, it allowed me to deliver vaginally, which is what I really wanted.*
>
> —ABIGAIL A., NEW MOM

- **Vocalize**. Breathing is great, but it's not going to get you through labor. (The last time you were hanging pictures and accidentally hit your thumb with the hammer, did you instinctively respond with "he-he whoo-whoo"? Probably not.) McMoyler Method utilizes the natural, human response to pain—minus the screaming. We recommend any kind of *productive* sound. Low, guttural sounds, moans, and sighs that come from deep inside and help move the contraction up and out of the body are effective and help labor progress. Screaming and high-pitched wailing are nonproductive and raise tension levels by registering with your brain as panic.

  To get an idea of the kind of moaning I'm talking about, think back to the last time you had some serious gastrointestinal trouble. Maybe it was in Mexico when you just couldn't resist buying a piece of fresh fruit from a street vendor. Or maybe it was the morning after a particularly raucous New Year's Eve party. Chances are you spent a lot of time in the bathroom, hunched over, making low moaning sounds. That's exactly the kind of productive sound that will help you cope with uterine contractions.

> *I wasn't that scared of labor because I had in my mind that I was going to get drugs! So I didn't really pay any attention to the coping strategies and pain-management techniques and kept thinking, "I'm so not going to need this." Well, the epidural didn't take completely, so there I was writhing in pain in the bed, hooked up to a million things, and I couldn't get up to walk around, or take a shower, etc. Fortunately, my husband kept his head and was able to keep me focused. He was great at telling me that we were on our way, the baby was coming, and that he loved me. Having him there to mirror the deep, guttural moaning was what got me through.*
>
> —BETSY R., NEW MOM

Medical Pain-Management Options

Your body is built to give birth, and McMoyler Method strongly supports natural childbirth. We believe that the combination of a strong support network and the noninvasive coping strategies discussed above provides a solid base to spring from, giving your body the time it needs to do the job on its own. I've worked with a lot of women who are 100 percent committed to giving birth exactly that way. And I've worked with plenty who are on the other end of the spectrum, what I call "parking-lot epidurals" (meaning you'd like to get hooked up to the medication before you even get out of your car). My goal here is to move you away from either extreme, to give you the information you need to help you make the choices that are right for you when the time comes. Again, I recommend that you give your body a fair shake to do what it was built to do before deciding on medical interventions.

> *For me, having an epidural was out of the question. I'm a vegetarian, I don't eat trans fats, and I never buy diet sodas with aspartame. I drink organic milk, eat organic produce, and won't allow PVC plastics in my house. And there was no way I was going to put any kind of drugs into my body. But after more than twenty hours of backbreaking labor, I was so exhausted I couldn't think straight. My doctor told me that I was heading for a cesarean. So I went with an epidural just to get some sleep. When I woke up, I was fully dilated and it was almost time to push. There's no question in my mind that having the epidural allowed my body to make progress and probably kept me from having a cesarean.*
>
> —HANA R., NEW MOM

Childbirth is completely unpredictable, and I can't emphasize this point enough: When it comes to pain, there's a big difference between coping and suffering. If labor stalls and you're experiencing the typical first-baby labor—long—and your mind and body are shot, something has to change. The good news is that here in the twenty-first century, there are viable, safe pain-management options: Pain medications take the edge off the peak of your contractions and make it easier for you to relax and recover between them. Epidurals numb the body from the waist down, replacing the pain with a feeling of pressure. (For many women, just knowing that there's a safety net out there in the form of *relief* gives them a sense of confidence that can significantly decrease the stress and strain of labor and make the journey more tolerable.)

The American College of Obstetricians and Gynecologists (ACOG) recently released a statement that you may find helpful as you consider your options: "Labor results in severe pain for many women. There is no other circumstance in which it is considered acceptable for a person to experience untreated severe pain, amenable to safe intervention, while under a physician's care. In the absence of a medical contraindication, maternal request is a sufficient medical indication for pain relief during labor. Pain management should be provided whenever it is medically indicated." You wouldn't get a root canal without exploring all the pain-management options. Why have a baby that way?

Two important things to consider: First, make sure you familiarize yourself with the nonmedical techniques in this chapter. Second, be open to the words of wisdom your nurses will have on the day of labor. Occasionally epidurals don't work completely. If that happens to you, you'll need some other coping mechanisms to help get you through.

> *I was definitely one of those "parking-lot epidurals." But after learning about the possible risks of medical intervention, I changed my mind and decided to go for a natural childbirth. . . . I'll keep you posted.*
>
> —TALIA B., EXPECTANT MOM

The decision to move from a no-intervention labor to a high-tech one is a big one and shouldn't be made lightly. Add in some people's political views on the subject and pressure from friends, family, and childbirth prep instructors to do whatever *they* think is best, and it can become complicated. So try to forget the politics and the pressure and instead, work with your health care professionals to make the decision that's best for *you*. There is absolutely no room in the birth process for guilt, regret, or feelings that you've failed. You're not going to win any prizes for having a natural childbirth. Deciding to use medical pain-management options is often the most responsible choice and does *not* make you bad parents.

There are two basic kinds of medical pain-management options. I want to give you a brief overview of both here, along with their advantages and disadvantages. You'll find a more detailed discussion in Chapter 6.

Analgesics. This category of drugs includes fast-acting narcotics (such as Demerol, Stadol, and Fentanyl) and tranquilizers (such as Phenergan or Vistaril). Administered intravenously, both act on your entire body and mind. They also cross the placental barrier and will temporarily decrease your baby's activity level. So while you're now able to at least rest in between contractions, your baby is sleeping. **Narcotics** don't relieve pain entirely, but what they can do is take the edge off the peak of the contraction. That, in turn, helps you release and let go in between contractions—even if it's only for a few minutes. On the downside, narcotics will most likely leave you feeling a little (or a lot) drowsy. They could cause some nausea and vomiting, and if given very close to delivery, the baby may need another medication to counteract the effects of the narcotic. **Tranquilizers** tend to decrease anxiety and, like narcotics, help you relax. When given together, tranquilizers increase narcotics' effectiveness and can alleviate some of the nausea and vomiting (if you have any). Used alone, though, they don't do anything at all for the pain.

Anesthetics. This category includes locals and epidurals. Both are delivered via injection, and the effect on the baby is minimal. **Locals** reduce or eliminate pain in a very specific part of the body (such as the perineum, when numbing it for an episiotomy or while repairing it after a tear). There are very few known side effects of local anesthesia, but again, the pain is relieved in a very small area. **Epidurals** combine a numbing agent with a narcotic and are typically injected into the lower back, in between the lumbar vertebrae. They relieve the pain (without sedation) in entire regions of the body, such as from the belly to the toes. They're typically given in the active phase of labor (when your cervix is dilated somewhere between 3 and 7 centimeters) and can actually assist your body in making progress by allowing for complete internal relaxation. On the downside, about 10 percent to 15 percent of the time, epidurals are less than completely effective. They may affect your ability to push and will typically keep you confined to your bed. That, in turn, could *increase* the length of your labor. There's also a *very* small chance of severe headaches, drop in blood pressure, or an allergic reaction to the medication. (Note that the McMoyler Method stance on this is that epidurals do not need to inhibit pushing; with the nurse and the partner as a cheering section, many, many women push babies out with an epidural on board.)

Advances in Epidural Technology

Today, about half of all babies are born to women who have had an epidural. In some parts of the country, it's as high as 80 percent, which is why I want to spend a little extra time talking about them.

Before epidurals were developed, there were spinals, which required the anesthesiologist to puncture the *dura,* the membrane that surrounds the spinal cord. If spinal fluid leaked out, you'd get a terrible headache. Spinals were almost always used very late in labor, just before delivery.

With epidurals, the anesthesiologist's needle is not intended to puncture the dura, which means fewer headaches. (Today, if the new mom *does* develop a headache, there's an immediate remedy available in the form of a simple procedure called a "blood patch.") The first generation of epidurals numbed women so much that they were confined to their beds and couldn't feel when to push. That sometimes lengthened labor and may have resulted in additional cesareans or assisted deliveries (using forceps or vacuum extraction).

Over the years, science has refined epidurals to such a degree that the result is a "walking epidural," named because most (though not all) women retain enough muscle control to get out of bed and walk around. Being mobile and still able to feel her contractions and when to push definitely is an advantage. Although these walking epidurals (sometimes called intra-thecal) are quickly gaining in popularity, they're not yet available everywhere.

Another new innovation is PCEA (patient-controlled epidural anesthesia). The anesthesiologist inserts the epidural catheter and starts pumping a very low flow of medication. The patient can increase the amount of medication she gets (up to preprogrammed maximums) by simply pushing a button. What's interesting is that in most cases, the patient gives herself less medication than she would have received with a standard epidural. Patients who feel in control and know that relief is nearby often don't feel the need to use it as much. Like walking epidurals, PCEA isn't available in every hospital, so check with your doctor or midwife to find out what your options are.

> *I way, way underestimated how much labor would hurt. I was literally screaming with each contraction. I held off on the epidural because I'm petrified of needles. But after a while I stopped caring and just wanted the pain to end any way possible. When the anesthesiologist came in I didn't even feel it when he put the needle in. About twenty minutes later I was feeling fantastic. If that anesthesiologist would have asked me to run away with him I would have done it on the spot (just kidding).*
>
> —ERIN D., NEW MOM

THE TRUTH BEHIND EPIDURALS

There's a lot of misinformation out there about epidurals. Here are a few of the common myths—and the reality you're less likely to hear about.

Myth: Epidurals lengthen labor and lead to cesareans and instrument-assisted births.

Reality: Although this may have been true as recently as ten years ago, new research is coming out every day that challenges these claims. Several recent studies have found that women who have epidurals are no more likely than unmedicated women to have a cesarean or need an assisted birth (using vacuum extraction or forceps).[1] Other studies have shown that epidurals may actually help labor progress by interrupting the fear-tension-pain cycle and allowing her to rest from head to toe.

Interestingly, there's a much stronger connection between perceived pain, long labors, and medical interventions. Women who rate their pain as "excruciating" or "horrible"—particularly early on in labor—are more likely to have cesareans, and twice as likely to have an instrument delivery, than women who perceive less pain. The attitude among women and childbirth educators who see only one way to give birth is narrow and rigid and doesn't allow for flexibility to make decisions based on each woman's individual needs and unique labor. Researchers have analyzed data from women whose epidural medication was dialed back near the pushing stage, in order to increase sensation. The results indicate that labors were not shorter and there were no fewer instrument deliveries. The only thing that changed was that women reported being in more pain.[2]

> *I've been a labor and delivery nurse for fifteen years and have seen it all. In my opinion, natural childbirth is the best and safest way to go, hands down. I don't think interventions are evil, it's just that I think they should be a last resort. When a patient has an epidural or some other pain medication, there are risks involved, risks that she should fully explore before making her decision.*
>
> —LISBETH Z., LABOR AND DELIVERY NURSE

Myth: Women who have had an epidural are more likely to have long-term back pain than women who had other forms of relief.

Reality: Another chicken-and-egg question. Back pain after a vaginal delivery can happen, but be careful where you place the blame. Is the culprit the pregnancy? The epidural? The birth itself? Throughout pregnancy the muscles and ligaments in your low back were continuously stretching in order to accommodate the growing uterus. That can result in some postpartum pain. During delivery, the descending baby can put a tremendous amount of painful pressure on your low back. And if you have an epidural, you may experience some residual tenderness at the spot where the anesthesiologist inserted the needle and catheter. The bottom line: Epidural-related postpartum back pain is the exception, not the rule.

Myth: The laboring woman's cervix has to be at least 4 centimeters dilated before an epidural can be used.

Reality: That used to be the recommendation of ACOG (American College of Obstetricians and Gynecologists). However, they recently came out with this revised policy: "Maternal request is a sufficient indication for epidural analgesia during labor and it should not be denied on the basis of cervical dilatation."

Myth: Women who have epidurals have trouble breastfeeding.

Reality: Several recent studies have found no significant difference in breastfeeding rates between women who had epidurals and those who didn't.[3] If, however—and this is a big *if*—epidurals do have an effect on a newborn's ability to latch on to the breast, that's something we need to deal with *after* the birth. I don't believe that epidurals should be withheld based on a *potential* effect. Let's get you through labor and delivery first and deal with breastfeeding later. With help from a lactation consultant, almost all babies will end up successfully breastfeeding. (See Chapter 6 for more on lactation consultants.)

Talking the Talk—and Then Talking Some More

Because the issue of pain is such a huge one to most expectant couples, we recommend that you have a series of conversations.

1. Ask your OB to explain all of your pain-management options, medical and nonmedical, that are applicable to the

hospital where you are delivering. Questions might include, "Will you be supportive if I want to have an unmedicated birth?" "How soon and/or how late will you allow me to have an epidural?" "Do they have walking epidurals at our hospital?"

2. Once you've got the information you need, you and your partner should sit down and talk about your thoughts and preferences—if he doesn't know them, he can't possibly be your advocate.
3. As soon as you're admitted to the hospital, you'll want to begin having ongoing conversations with the nursing staff and continue them throughout your labor. Discussing all your options with them while things are still relatively calm will save you time and aggravation later on. And remember, these are conversations, not obligations; keep your options open, and make your decisions along the way.

Conversation Starters for Conversation #2

1. Imagine a pain-management scale where one extreme is the "parking-lot epidural" and the other is "low- to no-intervention delivery" (meaning you really want to do the whole thing under your own steam). Where are you? The result of this discussion should be a statement like, "Honey, as soon as we get into our labor and delivery room, please tell our nurse where I am on the scale and ask her to support us in avoiding interventions/to get me my epidural as soon as humanly possible."
2. Spend some time talking about other occasions when you've felt extreme pain. How old were you when it happened? What caused the pain? Was there anything you or

someone else did that *helped?* Was there anything you or someone else did that made it worse?

3. I realize that it's going to be tough to have a productive conversation about how you're going to respond to something you've never experienced before. For that reason, I suggest that at least once a week, the two of you do the ice test that I describe on page 61. That will give you an opportunity to practice coping with and responding to intense discomfort.

CHAPTER

3

Why Your Husband Is the Most Important Person in the Delivery Room (Other than You)

WHAT YOU'LL LEARN IN THIS CHAPTER:

- How McMoyler Method dads are better prepared to be fully present throughout labor and delivery
- The difference between McMoyler Method dads and the traditional childbirth class dads
- Two critical things your husband needs to know about labor and delivery
- How your partner's involvement in labor and delivery sets the stage for becoming a family
- Getting even the most reluctant dad involved

ONE WAY OR another, you're going to have your baby. What remains to be seen is your husband's role in the process. As we've discussed, McMoyler Method dads are front and center. But what does that mean? What does a front-and-center dad do? What does he know that non–McMoyler Method dads don't?

To answer those questions, let me paint a picture of a fairly typical labor and delivery scenario to illustrate how a twenty-first-century dad differs from one who's taken a more traditional childbirth class.

Scenario 1: The Twentieth-Century Dad

It All Starts When Mom's Water Breaks . . .

The first thing he does is ask his wife for the doctor's phone number. While he's waiting for her to find it, he calls his mother and mother-in-law, and the neighbor lady next door, tells them the water broke, and asks them what to do now. When his wife returns with the phone number, he places the call to the doctor, who asks some general questions about when it happened, the color of the fluid, and so on. He is not sure that he knows the answers, so he'll have to get the information and call right back.

Arriving at the Hospital . . .

He is tentative, intimidated, and more than a little nervous (so is she). He's been through the classes, but they didn't talk about the parking situation. So he drops his wife off at the emergency room entrance and goes to park the car.

The Couple Arrive in Their Birthing Room

Dad hauls in the three large pieces of luggage, filled with a week's worth of clothing, as well as tennis balls, Coke cans, and a rolling pin for back massage. He hugs her and kisses her, asks her if everything's okay, and heads down to the cafeteria to grab a bite to eat. When he gets back, he checks in again, then heads out to the waiting room and nervously watches television with a few other expectant fathers who've gathered there. He checks in on her every little while, just to make sure everything is okay.

As Active Labor Begins . . .

The nurse comes down to the waiting room to say that his wife needs him. He is caught off-guard when he gets to his wife's room, as she is struggling with the contractions, which are now stronger. He does what he can to help out—he holds her hand, tries to use those breathing patterns, and brings her ice cream. He's feeling an increased sense of anxiety about what's happening. He's also a little put off by how messy this is getting; he does his best to give his wife privacy during the pelvic exam and tries to step away from the bed.

As Labor Progresses . . .

He's starting to get really concerned about the amount of pain his wife is in. She's not looking good at all, and he wishes someone would come in and do something. As labor intensifies, he feels more and more helpless. He tries to talk to his wife during contractions but this is irritating her. He is feeling helpless, and that he's in the way; he can feel the level of tension rising in the room and doesn't know what to do about it.

The Pain Intensifies and the Medical Team Suggests Some Medication or an Epidural

He now finds himself in a quandary. Clearly something needs to change—the breathing patterns they learned in class aren't working—but he's worried that the medication will hurt his baby. Plus he wants her to be able to follow the birth plan as much as possible.

He has questions but doesn't know where to begin, and he's suspicious that they might be trying to impose an intervention for their own convenience.

Overall, Dad Feels . . .

For this father, labor and birth are the means to an end—Mom has the baby, and their life as a family has begun. Dad feels like a spectator—a fish out of water. Mom is in labor and he has no idea what do. He's disappointed in himself for not being able to do more. Feeling useless is not high on his list . . . he ends up waiting in the chair over by the window.

Mom Feels . . .

She wants him there, really needs him, but he looks panicked. She feels a little embarrassed that her husband is seeing her in such a complete mess, physically and emotionally. She's wondering how on earth other women have coped with all this and is starting to think it would be better to just knock her out, wake her when it's over. . . .

Doesn't sound like a particularly inspiring experience, does it? Not only is it not great, it's simply not necessary. We are sure that last century the babies were as loved and cherished as this century; the difference is that the approach and attitude have changed.

Scenario 2: The Twenty-First Century Dad in Labor

McMoyler Method dads:

- Know to use vocalization to help her get through contractions
- Remind her to release and let go in between contractions
- Understand that verbal words of reassurance and encouragement are imperative
- Know a variety of ways to help labor progress and enhance coping (we cover these in detail in Chapter 4)
- Rely on and trust the health care team, and make decisions with their help
- Know that a variety of options are available for pain management

It All Starts When Mom's Water Breaks . . .

He takes a few minutes to gather the information he knows they'll ask for when he calls the hospital: color of the fluid, how much came out, what time it happened, whether his wife is having contractions, and whether the baby is moving around. Then he grabs the phone number off the refrigerator and makes the call.

Arriving at the Hospital . . .

They arrive feeling a sense of anticipation and relatively confident, knowing what the next steps are. He remembers from the tour of the hospital where to park on the weekend versus weekday, double parks near the entrance to Labor and Delivery, takes her upstairs, gets her settled, and then quickly moves the car.

The Couple Arrive in Their Labor Room

When he gets back to the room, he's carrying the three small duffel bags they brought from home: one for his wife, one for him, and one with a few things for the baby. He helps his wife out of her clothes and into a hospital gown. While she's in the bathroom, he double-checks that the camera has batteries, turns off his cell phone, and puts some breath mints on the bedside table and a few more in his pants pocket for good measure. Then he locates the linen closet in their room for extra hospital gowns, pillows, and washcloths.

When the nurse comes back in, he takes a few minutes to introduce himself, and he and his wife talk with her about their goals for the labor (avoiding interventions versus epidural ASAP). He asks where the pantry is and whether it's okay for him to get anything he needs for his wife. Will it be okay to get out of the bed in about an hour or so? Does she know where he can find a rocking chair to bring into their room? He heads off to get supplies, fills the sports bottle they brought from home with grape juice, water, and ice. He brings a little extra ice back to the room for cold compresses later. He asks at the nurses' station where the warmer is in case they need one of those big bath blankets to wrap her up in when she gets out of the shower.

Even though they took the hospital tour, this place is taking on a whole new meaning. . . .

As Active Labor Begins

His adrenaline is starting to flow as his wife's contractions intensify. Between contractions he tells her that she's doing really well, and rubs her down with the cold compresses. As the contractions get stronger, there's an increase in bodily fluids. The nurse comes in and he helps her change his wife's hospital gown and the under pads that she has been sitting on; he sees a lot more of the bloody show now—pretty messy, but he remembers that this is a sign of progress.

When the nurse comes back in to do a pelvic exam, he stands at the head of the bed, reminding her to breathe slowly and steadily, not to hold her breath, and to drop her shoulders and unclench her teeth. After the exam, they ask the nurse about the exam. Is the baby's head in a position that will help labor progress? Is the cervix dilating?

He remembers that as the contractions get stronger, they come closer together, and that's definitely happening. Luckily, the nurse stays with them and helps him get nose-to-nose with his wife. He mimics the nurse and moans repeatedly to remind his wife to do the same. At the end of the contraction he takes a deep breath and exhales loudly with her. Then he helps her to let her body go, to release and let go of every muscle, to close her eyes and rest. The nurse is monitoring the baby's heart rate and telling them that everything looks good.

As Labor Progresses . . .

He's starting to wonder whether these contractions could possibly get any stronger. . . .

The nurse helps him move his wife into the bathroom, where she sits on the toilet for a few minutes, until they get the shower ready. He gets his swim trunks on and he and the nurse help move her into the warm shower. He holds her in a slow-dance position, the water running down her back. During each contraction, he helps her focus, he does the moaning and tells her to follow his lead, to stay with him, that he has her, that she's okay. After the contraction, he gets her situated under the water again, and for the hundredth time has her let go and catch that rest between contractions. The next contraction starts and they do it all over again. The nurse pops in about every ten minutes to check on them.

The Pain Intensifies and the Medical Team Suggests Some Medication or an Epidural

He and the nurse tell her that she's done a great job, that she shouldn't be hard on herself, and that it's time to consider other options. He is so relieved to have the health care team to rely on for what to do. They've seen this a million times. He just wants her to get some relief and rest.

Dad Feels . . .

He is not a spectator; he can't imagine being in the waiting room or watching TV. He knows he's done everything in his power to help her. He's in awe of how hard she's been working through this; now it's time to switch gears.

He feels pretty overwhelmed; it looks excruciating. He's grateful for how great the nurses have been. He's amazed by his wife's strength, and relieved that she's made enough progress to get some help with the pain. If this seems surreal to him, he's trying to imagine how it must feel for her.

Overall, Mom Feels . . .

1. Relieved to be in the hospital, where she has options
2. Glad to have such great nurses—they're a Godsend
3. Like she needs her husband now more than ever. She can't imagine going through this without him. He is keeping her focused and calm. Every time she feels she's going to lose it, he brings her back. She'll never forget how he stayed with her no matter what was going on.

DadBox

You need to understand two things.

1. Childbirth is not a spectator sport.
2. It is, however, an extreme sport for her, and she needs you to be involved.

Think of labor as a wild, whitewater river. The woman you love is about to go through some pretty rough rapids. It could last four hours, or twenty-four. No one knows for sure, but it's going to happen. She's got enough to do just staying inside the boat, but she's also afraid of losing control of the raft and of the pain she'll go through. She needs to be able to let go of her superwoman complex and accept the idea of turning the steering over to someone else—that would be you. She also needs to feel confident that you've brought the life vests and crash helmets, looked at the map, will be with her through every turn, and know how to rely on the professionals for backup.

You need to be able to help navigate your wife to a place where she can check her social graces at the door, let go of her inhibitions, and let her body do its work. It's the place where labor progresses more effectively, a place she'll never get to if she feels scared or alone.

You love her and can provide unconditional support unlike anyone else in the building. Your encouragement, reassurance, and help making decisions along the way are essential—no one can take your place. But if the going gets tough to the point that you need to call for backup, they're there. Your nurses and doctors are not afraid of her pain. When they see something that looks and feels beyond intense, they see it as a good thing: It's called making progress—it means the baby is coming.

Getting Dad Involved

Most expectant couples these days have the following in common: a desire to be knowledgeable about the birth process and to know how to care for their new baby. The problem is that, like many expectant dads, your husband may not be exactly sure what to do and is worried that he'll get in the way. This is where things can get a little tricky. If you just sit back and wait for him to step in, you could be waiting a long time. So if you want him to be there, actively involved, you're going to need to come right out and say so. There are two ways to go about this; you can do one or both of the following.

1. The direct approach. During a calm moment, the two of you sit down together and you actually say the words, "Honey, I need you, I love you, and I can't do this without you." Unfortunately, the cultural message that labor and delivery is "women's work" dies hard, so don't be shy about telling him now that you are counting on him, that all you want and need are his love and support to see you through this.
2. The indirect approach. You hand him a copy of this book, which tells him why he's so important (in this chapter—especially the DadBox on page 51) and gives him the knowledge he needs and the steps he can take to be able to participate throughout labor and delivery (in the following chapter). You should also pick up a copy of my co-author's book *The Expectant Father,* which will help him stay involved throughout the entire pregnancy.

Not all expectant dads truly want to be as involved as we'd like, and some may not respond to either of the approaches described above. I remember one guy who sat at the head of the bed and simply held his wife's hand—that was all he could do. Another, who had fainting issues, called into the labor room from the *waiting* room—that was as close as he could get. And then there was the dad who burst through the door, floating on air with happiness *after* the baby was born—based on his cultural and religious beliefs, he simply couldn't be an actual part of the birth. I have no doubt that all of these guys turned out to be great dads.

If you think that your husband is a potential low-involvement dad, remember that communication is key. Encourage him to talk about what's bothering or worrying him, and listen respectfully. Trying to force the issue or disregard his personal limits won't work. The good news is that many, many men surprise themselves on the day of labor by moving way beyond their own comfort zone.

WHAT THE EXPERTS SAY

This book is designed to be very practical and hands-on. This chapter's focus is on the simple fact that your husband isn't just a nice-to-have kind of guy—he's essential to the process. In addition to what we know from McMoyler graduates, here's what the research shows.

Starting at the beginning, dads who have learned about labor and who know how to participate tend to be more actively involved, and their wife's experiences tend to be better.[1] That's exactly what's coming in the next chapter. And when labor partners (including fathers) have learned a lot about pain control, women have shorter labors and are less likely to have epidurals.[2]

As you can imagine, women whose partners are supportive during labor and delivery feel more in control of the birth process (meaning that they understand what's happening and are participating in decision-making). They report experiencing less pain and have more positive childbirth experiences.[3,4]

Dad's level of involvement can be a good predictor of how involved he'll be later on. Being at the birth, plus getting the chance to spend a lot of time interacting with the baby right after birth, may stimulate such nurturing behavior as feeding and diaper changing.[5] It also increases the chance that Dad will come to well-child pediatrician visits later on.[6]

Your husband's involvement before the baby's birth can also have a big impact on the kind of mother you become. Women whose husbands are supportive during labor have a more positive attitude toward motherhood.[7]

Time to Lose the Cape

In today's fast-paced world, women are expected to do it all, to be superheroes—manage their schedule, their finances, their homes, their bodies, their vacations, and just about everything else. Once they get pregnant, though, everything changes. These completely in-control women find themselves in a situation where they're not in charge anymore. Things are happening to their body that they have little if any control over. They've heard from their friends about how intense contractions are. They worry that they won't be able to manage the pain or that they'll behave so primitively, be so out of control, do something so socially unacceptable that they'll have to move out of town. Yikes.

And as they look around at their friends who now have kids, it starts to dawn on them that raising a family is a tough job. For today's competent, in-charge women, the prospect of being so out of control can be frightening. So they move into overdrive, reading books, taking courses, spending hours on the Internet, hoping to find some way to regain control of their lives before the dreaded labor starts.

I hate to be the one to break the news to you, but it's important to put a reality-based spin on this: If you don't pack up your Superwoman cape right now, pronto, you're in for a rude awakening. No matter how many books and articles you read or classes you take, you'll still want to have an unconditional source of support, someone who loves you from your head to your toes who will provide a presence throughout the entire process.

Dad as Doula

In the past few years, it has become very trendy in some circles to hire a *doula* (a female labor companion) to provide the kind of help I'm talking about. In principle, the concept is a good one, and I've worked with some wonderful doulas who made important contributions and really helped. Many of you will go on to hire doulas, and that will be the right decision for your needs and your situation. I do, however, want to address why the doula question can be a little more complicated.

To start with, the vast majority of doulas are unlicensed and have no medical training. I'll talk about that in more detail in Chapter 7. The bigger issue, though, is that you already have the best doula you can get: your husband. He knows you better and loves you more than anyone else does. He knows your fears and your desires, and because he has a big stake in the outcome, no one can be a better or more committed advocate for you than he will. (Even the nurses, as great as they are, do not actually love you. Remember that your husband will be there for you and the baby long after the doula goes home.)

At the end of the day, here's McMoyler Method's stand on doulas:

- Your husband can be your primary support person. If you really want additional support, consider asking a dear friend or family member, someone who will be unconditionally supportive of you, your husband, and your decisions.
- If you have the money to spend on a doula ($500–$2,000), consider using it for postpartum care instead. With all the attention paid to labor and delivery, it's sometimes easy to forget that that's just the beginning. You'll have plenty of people to take care of you while you're at the hospital; home is a different story—especially if you don't have a nearby network of close friends and family. Keep in mind that mothers and mothers-in-law are not always the best

choice, and their help can sometimes come with a high price tag in terms of stress—and you'll have plenty of that already. (No offense intended here to grandparents—we happen to think that most of them are saints. There will, however, be times when relatives will not be the best choice, so choose carefully and get the support that's right for you.)

DadBox

Having the Baby Is Just the Beginning

Being an active, engaged participant throughout labor and delivery is a wonderful opportunity—and will transform the two of you forever. By the time your baby is born, you'll have:

- Been with your wife every step of the way
- Moaned and groaned with her and guided her through a variety of positions designed to help her cope with the pain
- Helped her uncurl her body and relax between contractions, never letting her forget that you love her
- Gotten the nurses there in a hurry when you needed their help
- Helped make decisions and reassured her she was doing the right thing
- Been the first person to hold your baby
- Spent three nights on an uncomfortable hospital cot and hopped up every time a nurse came through the door to watch what they do and to have her watch you practice diaper changing, temperature taking, checking the cord, clearing the nose with the bulb syringe, and so on

Before *and* after the baby is born, one of the most important objectives will be to encourage your wife to keep her Superwoman cape in storage. When new families have reasonable expectations and give themselves ample time to adjust to the new little human in the house, they do much better. When moms hang on to the idea that they can forge ahead with their prebaby life, schedule, and activities, they're setting themselves up for a crash landing. Continue providing support and/or running interference at home; I'm a firm believer that if new moms are given permission to slow down and ease into their new role, the incidence of postpartum depression can be reduced. Remember the old adage: One of the most important things a father can do is love the mother.

CHAPTER

4

Game Plan for Dads: What *You're* Going to Be Doing during Labor and Delivery

WHAT YOU'LL LEARN IN THIS CHAPTER:

- Everything you need to know about your role during labor and delivery
- How to prepare yourself *during* pregnancy for the big day
- All about bodily fluids—what goes in and what's coming out
- McMoyler Maneuvers—active approaches to increase her ability to cope
- The PURRR test: the checklist confirming that you're doing everything you can for her

Okay, Dad, You're On!

We'd like to think that you've been reading this book along with your wife. If you're just joining us, we want to make sure that you get this message loud and clear: Aside from your wife, *you* are the most important person in the labor and delivery room. No one expects you to handle any of the medical issues that will come up—the doctors and nurses will take care of all that. What I want to do here is underscore your role and give you the information you need to help navigate through labor and delivery and to be a strong advocate for her. This is not to overlook the medical staff—you will need them. However, you have *the* closest connection to your wife and baby, and with that comes a source of strength and trust that she will need.

The bottom line is this: Regardless of how your baby is born, you are essential to the birth process, and no one can take your place. Your presence and unconditional love and support make a *huge* difference in your wife's ability to do this. For most of the rest of this chapter, I'm going to tell you exactly what your role is. But before we launch into what to do during labor and delivery, let's talk about what you're doing in the months and weeks *before* you jump in the car and head for the hospital.

Prenatal Prep

The seventh month of pregnancy is when the real countdown begins. So start getting your game plan established now, while you've still got a lifestyle that's somewhat predictable.

Plan to set aside a specific time once a week when the two of you can commit to focusing for ten to fifteen minutes. I know you think you're busy, but you don't know the meaning of the word yet. Plus, we consider the birth of your baby the biggest event of your life, so take these suggestions to heart. Pick a date and time and put it into whatever calendar system you both use. Make it part of your regular routine. For example, every Saturday morning while we're having coffee in bed (not too many more of those days left), or every Monday when we go out for Thai food. You get the idea.

To jump-start and guide your discussions, we've developed a list using the mnemonic HEALTHY MOM AND BABY. You won't be able to get through the entire list in one sitting, and some items will take longer than others, so take your time. The more conversations you have like this, the clearer you'll be with each other and the better prepared you'll be to communicate with the health care team on the actual day of delivery.

> *I'll admit that I resisted going through all these exercises and discussions—they definitely seemed a little silly at first. But having done them, I realize that they brought up issues and areas that we had not considered. I found out that my husband had a lot more concerns about the whole thing than I was aware of. It also prompted him to do a few things while we were pregnant that I'm sure he wouldn't have made time for otherwise. (The weekend away was a big surprise and turned out to be our last getaway before the baby was born.)*
>
> —FRANCESCA R., NEW MOM

Have conversations about the birth. How does each of you imagine that day will go? This conversation will take place more than once, as your thinking will be influenced by everything you read, every movie you see, and so on.

Explain to each other at least one of your concerns about the birth. Write these down so you can bring them up at your next prenatal visit or childbirth class.

Ask your parents about their birth experiences. What was it like the day you were born? Ask them to also jot down their memories in an e-mail or letter. These are great to have as a keepsake.

Leave a note for your partner. Something short and sweet, such as "I love you and can't wait to meet our baby," or "You look gorgeous—see you tonight." Find new places to put these notes.

Under her pillow, in his briefcase, on the dashboard of the car, taped to the bathroom mirror, folded inside the newspaper . . .

Telephone her in the middle of the day. This is a brief, unexpected call, something like, "How are you?" "How's the baby?" "Meet me for dinner at our favorite place," "Be ready at 7:00. I have a surprise for you."

Help her tackle the long baby to-do list. For example, do some research into strollers and cribs, make an appointment to get your car seat properly installed (see the sidebar below for more), or go to cpsc.org to check into any recent baby-product recalls.

Yogurt smoothies to die for. Become an expert when it comes to making her a healthy snack or breakfast on the run. Buy organic, nonfat yogurt and frozen fruit—bananas, strawberries, blueberries, mango—any kind she likes.

TIME TO TAKE A (CAR) SEAT

To take your baby home from the hospital you must have a rear-facing infant car seat installed in your car. When looking at car seats, consider one with a detachable base (the base stays attached to the car, while the seat part comes out with you). That way you put the baby into the seat before leaving and you just snap the seat into the base. Do yourself a favor and learn how to properly install the car seat before you get to the hospital. There's a right way and a wrong way and it can be a little tricky the first few times. Many police and fire departments will give you a brief tutorial for free. In some cases, they'll actually install it for you. Check out seatcheck.org or nhtsa.org for locations and other car seat–related tips, and car-safety.org for information on ratings. (In the extremely unlikely case that your wife is in active labor in the car and needs to lie down in the backseat, you'll have to uninstall the car seat and reinstall it later.)

Moaning. The human response to pain is to make some kind of sound, which is often accompanied by clenching the teeth and constricting the throat (see Chapter 2 for an in-depth discussion). Learning to make *productive* sounds will take a little practice. Start by humming for about five seconds. Now unhinge your jaw and let it drop open. Next, open up your throat muscles and let out a long, slow "heeeeeeeeeeee." Take another breath and let out a long, slow "hawwwwwwwwwwwwww." Practice this once a day. You can do it alone, in the shower, when you're on the toilet, driving, or whenever. Go ahead, let your imagination run wild. . . .

THE COLD FACTS

When I first began teaching McMoyler Method, I found myself looking for a way to simulate the discomfort of a contraction so I could have my students practice moaning in a more realistic way. So I came up with what I call the ice test. Here's what you do:

- Dump some ice cubes into a bowl and set your kitchen timer for ninety seconds.
- Have your wife pick up as many ice cubes as she can hold, and squeeze.
- Start the timer.
- While she's squeezing the ice, you get up close, nose to nose, and do some of that in-your-face mirroring.
- Have her inhale deeply and exhale loudly.
- For the next twenty seconds or so, have her keep breathing slowly as she rides the "contraction" up.
- Now you're at the peak. Switch to moaning and keep it up for the next forty seconds. Talk to her, encourage her with phrases like, "Keep it up, you can do this, follow me, let your jaw go, that's it . . ."
- When you've got twenty to twenty-five seconds left, start slowing her breathing down as the "contraction" subsides.
- Now have her take one more big, deep breath and exhale audibly.
- Turnabout is fair play, so set the timer for another ninety seconds. But this time, *you* squeeze the ice and your wife mirrors for you. I'm sure you'll find this surprisingly uncomfortable—and challenging.

Order flowers, for no reason at all. (Hint: There's no reason you can't do this more than once.)

Make appointments to interview pediatricians. You need to have selected a doctor for your baby *before* the baby is born. Don't put this one off for too long. Some pediatric groups don't schedule actual interviews—they simply don't have time. In this case, plan to visit the practice you are considering to at least meet the front office staff and ask some individual questions. Your OB/midwife, family, and friends are excellent sources of referrals.

COUNTIN' KICKS

A simple—and very important—way to check on your baby's well-being during the last few months of pregnancy is to do kick counts. After your wife has had something to eat and drink and can sit down for a bit, she (or the two of you together) needs to count the number of kicks until you get to five. This usually happens within a few minutes (babies generally respond quickly to food/fluid and Mom getting off her feet), but it could take as long as an hour. If you don't get enough of those reassuring kicks by then, call her OB or midwife. She may need to go into the office or the Labor and Delivery unit for some monitoring. Kick counts should be done once every day during the pregnancy (ask your OB/midwife when she wants you to begin) and once an hour during labor at home.

Apply counterpressure to her low back. This is a massage with the heel of your hand, anywhere from the low back to the tailbone. You can either press firmly in one place or make circles with the heel of your hand. Ask her which she prefers, high or low, firm or stationary; what feels good while she's pregnant is likely to change during labor . . . keep inquiring.

Name your baby. There are dozens of name books out there, and literally hundreds of Web sites that feature name dictionaries. The fact is that you don't actually need to make this decision until just before you leave the hospital, so don't stress too much.

Dad's night out. Go out with a few male friends who have kids. Spend some time over a beer picking their brains to get their tips on what works and what doesn't. Women tend to be much better at this but given a chance, men have plenty to say on the subject.

Buy lollipops for labor. For a few reasons, sucking on lollipops is a popular labor and delivery pastime; they provide a bit of sugar and stimulate the salivary glands—her mouth will get dry over time. Shop online for sweet *and* sour; they seem to be the favorite.

Ask around your neighborhood for daycare and babysitter recommendations. It's never too soon to do this. Finding the right caregivers can take quite a while.

Buy the grandparents a small gift. A frame for that first baby photo is nice. Include a note that acknowledges *them* and their new roles as grandparents. This is a good opportunity to think about how you want to approach the idea of getting support from them after the baby comes. Do you want them coming immediately? To the hospital, or later to your home? Do they stay in a hotel or with you?

Year of the baby's birth. Start your baby's scrapbook by clipping out some front-page headlines, weather, politics, where we lived when you were born, and so on. Although archiving all these things online is nice, there's something special about having an actual book to hold. That way you can include actual artifacts like the baby's security bracelets.

KNOW YOUR SURROUNDINGS

If you haven't already done so, take a tour of the hospital. Where's the parking lot? Is valet parking available? Where do you enter the hospital? Some have different entrances open, depending on the day of the week or time of day. Where are the elevators in relation to the hospital entrances?

On the day you check into the hospital, take a few minutes to survey the room and the labor and delivery unit. You're going to be in that room for hours and hours, so go ahead and open up the cabinets to see where they keep the washcloths, gowns, bath blankets, extra pillows. Most of the time the nurse will get these for you, but if she's also busy caring for other patients, understand that she may not be able to get them as quickly as you'd like them. While you're at it, try to find out where the wheeled stool is (for you to sit on), the shower, the nurse call button, and the controls for the electronic bed.

At eight months, continue working through the previous list and add in the following, using the words RELEASE AND LET GO:

Research grocery stores and restaurants that will deliver great food to you. This can be handy while you're busy expectant parents. It'll be a lifesaver after the baby arrives.

Enroll in an infant CPR/safety class. We highly recommend that you take this important class *before* the baby comes. Too many people intend to do this after the baby is born and never get around to it.

Laugh. Whether it's *I Love Lucy* or reruns of *Saturday Night Live,* or going to a comedy club, do the things that make you laugh. Humor is one of the best weapons for dealing with the stress that babies naturally create.

Exhale. When we're stressed or just concentrating, we have a tendency to hold our breath (it's a completely unconscious act—most of us have no idea we're doing it). Long, slow, deep breaths are best. Practice this a lot since she'll need to be reminded to do this at the beginning and end of every contraction.

Appoint a contact person who will update your friends and family with progress during labor. You're not going to want to field tons of calls while you're in labor, so ask your contact person to put together a phone tree.

Start packing. Your bags should be ready to go by thirty-six weeks. Most people bring way too much gear with them to the hospital. See pages 69–70 for our recommended packing lists for Mom, Dad, and Baby.

Expect her mood to fluctuate. Shifting hormones, an expanding belly, and a mind trying to prepare itself for a painful experience can wreak havoc with her emotions. Stay supportive; she needs your encouragement.

Apply to nursery schools. I know, I know, your baby isn't even born yet. In some areas the waiting lists start long before the babies arrive.

Notify friends and family that what you really want are gifts of food, not flowers. This can be a home-cooked meal or even a gift certificate for a favorite take-out place.

Discuss what happens if you end up having a cesarean birth. Will Dad go to the nursery with the baby or stay in the operating room with Mom? It is extremely helpful to have discussed this ahead of time; in a situation when a cesarean is unexpected, couples need to transition quickly to the new game plan. At least this has been considered in advance.

Listen to your body. Are you having contractions? Pressure in the low pelvis, an internal tightening, and your entire abdomen is hard as a rock? Many women will have what are called Braxton-Hicks contractions, which essentially are practice contractions (the uterus may fire off a contraction every now and then, perhaps four or five times a day). Real labor contractions develop a pattern, and over time the pattern of contractions will get stronger, longer, closer.

Elaborate on your labor and delivery goals. Do you want an epidural as soon as possible or do you want to avoid interventions? Dads, write this down so that *you* are clear about her desires.

Time contractions. Besides keeping track of how long they last, you'll also want to record how far apart they are, as measured from the beginning of one contraction to the beginning of the next. Partners, the first questions you'll be asked when you call the hospital to see if it's time to go are: "How often are they coming and how long are they lasting?"

Gifts for the hospital team. This is not a requirement, but I can tell you from experience that they really love it when you bring in a basket of chocolate chip cookies! We know you're busy, so it's not necessary to bring home-baked goodies—it's the thought that counts.

Outline your exit plan. Coffee pot off, lights on/off, neighbors covering the mail and newspapers, gas in the car, house secured, and so on. Outline your re-entry plan too: Make sure the house is ready to receive a new baby and recuperating mom; stock the laundry room and kitchen so when people offer to help you can send them in the right direction; and make sure you and your wife both know where you're going to keep all the baby supplies (diapers, wipes, clean clothes, and so on).

It's Showtime—Well, Almost

There are many concepts and phrases to become familiar with. The following are among the most important. Once labor starts, you'll be hearing them over and over. I also want to introduce you to some of the unexpected and unusual things—including a whole range of bodily fluids—you're going to be seeing between now and the time your baby is in your arms. One additional note: Some of the things you're going to be reading about are going to sound really bizarre (like demonstrating for your wife how to moan and groan, and spending a lot of time in the shower with her at the hospital). But believe me, when you're in the middle of it, it'll all seem necessary and important.

- **Stronger, longer, closer.** This has to do with contractions and is the key to telling whether your wife's labor is the real deal or false labor, and whether it's time to call the doctor and get ready to head to the hospital or time to fire up another DVD. True labor contractions will get stronger, last longer, and come closer together over time. False labor does not do this; there is no "pattern" of contractions with false labor.
- **In-her-face mirroring.** Don't waste time trying to have a rational conversation with a woman who's working through an intense contraction. She can't hear you! The best way to communicate with her is to physically show her what she needs to do. So get in front of her, make eye contact, and use your own body language to demonstrate how to unclench your jaw, relax your shoulders, open your hands, moan, rock, and so on. Watch the nurses in action; they know this approach inside and out.
- **Release and let go.** Unbeknownst to most people, it's as important to assist her *between* the contractions as it is to help her during them. When in severe pain, particularly pain that comes back again and again at predictable intervals (such as uterine contractions), it's natural to tense up right before each jolt and stay that way until the pain goes away. The problem is that staying tense between contractions, as we discussed in Chapter 2, feeds the fear-tension-pain cycle and makes it harder for her to cope. Helping her release her tension and let it go during the break between contractions allows her body to recover and her mind to center, and is the perfect time to remind her that she's okay and doing a good job.

- **Verbal anesthesia and emotional support.** Phrases like "you're doing fine," "great," wonderful," and so on go a long, long way toward keeping her focused and motivated through what is typically a long haul. (If first babies do anything, they take their sweet time being born.) The object here is to gently and steadily encourage and support her while letting her know you're there for the duration.
- **Up, walk, rock, change position.** Making this your mantra will help keep labor progressing. Being *upright* allows gravity to assist the baby to descend. *Walking* keeps her body in motion and maximizes the effect that *relaxin* (a hormone that does just that) can have on the pelvic joints. *Rocking* can help move a baby from a posterior presentation (aka "sunny side up") to a more desirable anterior position, helps the baby descend, and increases Mom's ability to release and let go between contractions. *Changing positions* at least every forty-five minutes keeps the body and mind from slipping into a mode called *habituation* (the struggle to continue to do something that is painful over a long period of time), where labor can stall. For some tested suggestions of what to do while you're encouraging your wife to get up and move around, see the section "McMoyler Maneuvers" below.

Bodily Fluids

One of the most curious parts of this whole labor and delivery process is how wet it is, so get your waders on. . . . Here are the most important ones. Some of this may make you (and possibly your wife) a little squeamish. So let's talk about what all those bodily fluids look like, what's normal, and what warrants a call to the doctor.

PACKING YOUR BAGS

You're not going on a six-month, around-the-world cruise, so let's keep things simple. Here are three short lists of hospital must-haves: one for Mom, one for you, one for the baby.

For Mom

- Two pairs of warm socks for labor (athletic type that she won't mind tossing out).
- Bathrobe, two short nighties, and slippers for postpartum. With all the bodily fluids coming, don't bring your nicest or newest.
- One or two pillows from home, in brightly colored pillowcases (to distinguish yours from the hospital's).
- Toiletries, just the basics (all women seem to overdo this one).
- Glasses. Contacts aren't good during labor. If she wears glasses, bring them.
- Jewelry: leave it and any other valuables at home.
- A favorite blanket or quilt for the postpartum room. Not a necessity, but it can really help personalize her bed.
- Loose-fitting clothes and comfortable shoes to wear home.

For You

- Your toiletries, swimsuit for labor, and a change of clothes.
- A small cooler with a few drinks, bottles of water, and snacks. Hospitals have cafeterias and you can sometimes dash out to pick yourself up something to eat when you need to.
- Breath mints. Lots. Your wife will smell your coffee breath the second you get off the elevator, and brushing your teeth is *not* good enough.
- Battery-operated CD or MP3 player and favorite music (the hospital may not allow you to plug things in).
- Camera with extra film, batteries, and memory cards.
- Calling card for long distance (many hospitals discourage the use of cell phones) and a few select numbers, including the person who will start spreading both progress in labor as well as the good news through the phone tree.
- Some cash.

- Your labor supplies:
  - Massage lotion or oil
  - Scrunchies for women with long hair
  - Handheld paper fan or a small battery-operated one
  - Sports bottle for fluids during labor
  - Lollipops
  - Lip balm

For Baby

- Car seat (see page 60)
- Outfit with feet so you'll be able to use the car seat harness
- T-shirt
- Blanket
- Knit hat or baby beanie

Mucous plug. Due to hormone shifts, a thick mucous plug develops in the cervix early in pregnancy. It protects the pregnant uterus from bacteria. Passing the mucous plug (which looks like a few tablespoons of egg white streaked with pinkish-brownish blood) is a major milestone—it means that you've got anywhere from a few hours to a few days before labor begins. (Although it's possible to go

MomBox

For some first-time moms, the mucous plug comes out in dribs and drabs, but more typically, there will be a little "event"—a surprise in their panties or a plop into the toilet. As your due date nears, you'll need to be able to tell the difference between increased vaginal discharge, urinary incontinence, leaking amniotic fluid, and the mucous plug. Sometimes that can be a lot to decipher. Please understand that there is no need to bring it with you to the hospital. I had a couple once who brought in the mucous plug in a little artichoke-heart jar, thinking that we would want to see it to be sure. Really and truly, all you have to do is describe it—we know what these things look like!

as long as a week without labor starting, most fall into the hours-to-days category.) Once the mucous plug is out, you're going to want to stay pretty close to home until you leave for the hospital. Please note, some women pass their mucous plug without noticing it, so don't be alarmed if yours is not the "event" we've described.

Amniotic fluid. When the amniotic sac that has been surrounding your baby for the past nine months or so ruptures on its own, fluid will come out. If the sac ruptures high up in the uterus, your wife will experience a trickle of fluid. If the rupture happens down low, she'll get a big gush. What's surprising to a lot of people is just how much amniotic fluid there is—sometimes it just seems to keep coming and coming and coming, which is actually true, since the placenta and the baby keep on manufacturing fluid until they're both delivered.

Sometimes this "water breaking" can cause contractions to begin; sometimes not. And about half the time, your doctor will end up doing an AROM (artificial rupture of membranes), which we call "snagging the bag," at the hospital. This simple procedure may help labor progress by allowing the baby's head to descend. AROM also provides the medical team with a valuable look at the color of the amniotic fluid. Discoloration of the fluid often indicates that the baby has passed *meconium*—its first stool. Meconium-stained fluid sometimes will require internal monitoring during labor and additional suctioning after delivery.

If you or your wife thinks her water has broken, call your OB or midwife right away. She'll ask you a number of questions, including the color, odor, amount, what time it happened, whether she's having contractions, and whether there has been any change in the baby's movements. So before you pick up the phone, make sure you know the answers to those questions. Depending on the answers, the doctor or midwife will tell you to head out for the hospital or to take it easy at home and check back in a few hours. If you're staying home, keep doing your kick counts. It's imperative to call if you "think" the water is leaking or if you "know" the water broke. Depending on your individual situation, the doctor or midwife will give you specific instruction.

MomBox

In a "gross rupture," meaning the amniotic sac breaks down near the baby's head, the amount of fluid that comes out can range from cups to quarts and there'll be no question about what happened. The kitchen floor (or wherever you were standing) has a puddle on it and your socks will be soaked. When you come into the hospital you'll be given huge saddle-size sanitary pads and some stretchy, one-size-fits-all panties to wear. This will allow you to move around without leaving a little trail behind you. With strong contractions, fluid will definitely be squeezed out, so from time to time the nurse will have to change the underpads hospitals use to catch the ever-increasing amount of fluids now exiting your body. Two pieces of advice: First, make sure you have plenty of maxi pads around the house—waiting until your water breaks to send your husband to get them is too late. Plus you'll need *a lot* of them postpartum. Second, if you haven't already done so, put a waterproof mattress pad on your bed. There's no guarantee, of course, that your water will break while you're in bed, but if any of that fluid gets into your mattress, you'll be shopping for a new one within a few weeks.

> *I was glad to be warned about certain things that would have caught me off-guard or grossed me out completely if I had not been prepared for them. When my wife's water broke, neither of us had any idea there would be so much fluid—it just about covered the bathroom floor. We called in, and the nurse asked me a bunch of questions about the fluid and told us to come in to get checked out.*
>
> —BOB J., NEW DAD

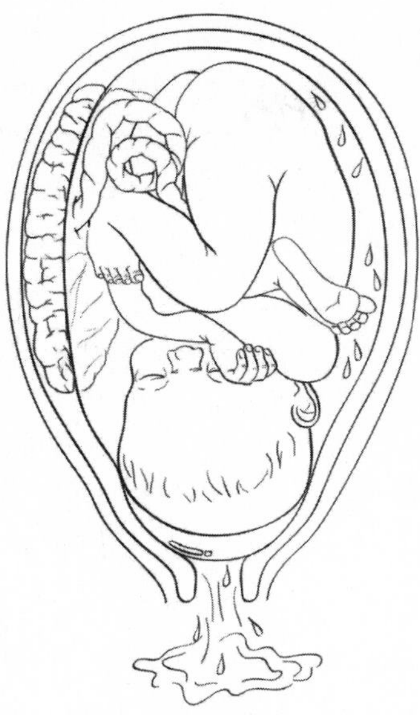

Spontaneous rupture:
high break

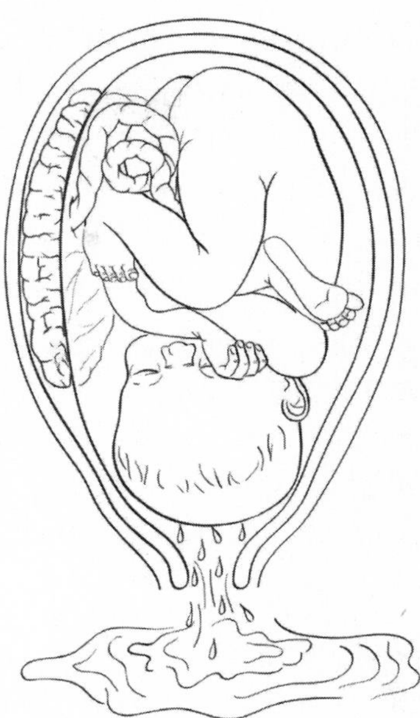

Spontaneous rupture:
low break

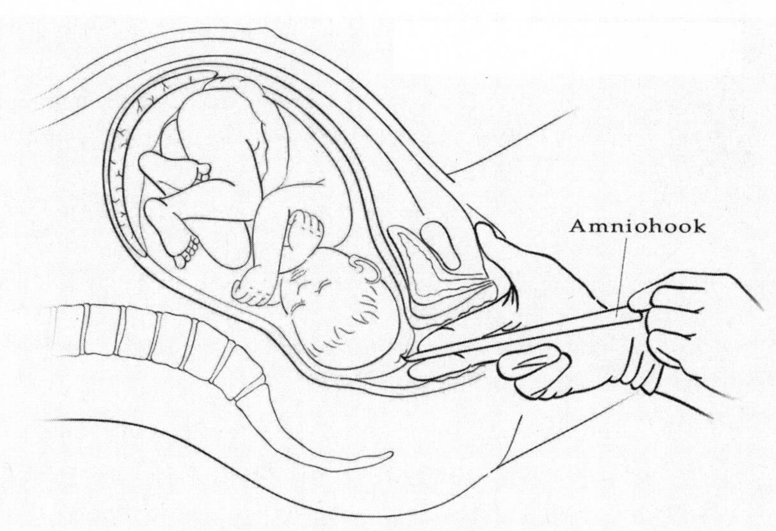

Artificial rupture—"snagging the bag"

Bloody show. Another important sign of progress. Some women may see a little of this at home, while others won't see it until they get to the hospital. Either way, if you don't know to expect it, it can be quite alarming. Bloody show occurs as a result of the cervical tissue stretching beyond its capacity. This stretching causes tiny lacerations, which bleed ever so slightly (small amounts of blood early on, more as labor progresses). When that blood mixes together with normal vaginal secretions and amniotic fluid, you'll get a little bit of pink on the toilet tissue after your wife empties her bladder. Bloody show is *not* heavy bleeding into the toilet bowl like the first day of a heavy period. If that happens, get her off the toilet and go immediately to the nearest hospital, as the placenta may be doing something that it shouldn't.

TIME TO GO?

Before you head to the hospital, make sure you do the following:

- Use the walk/talk test to determine whether the time is right. If your wife can't walk or talk during a contraction, that's a good indicator that this is serious labor.
- Always call either your OB/midwife or Labor and Delivery before leaving the house. They'll help you determine whether it's time to go and will begin preparing a labor room.
- If you're told to labor at home for a while, do kick counts (see page 62) until you arrive at the hospital.
- Consider the time of day, day of the week, distance to the hospital, and time you think it will take to get there.

Blood. There's going to be some, so prepare yourself. It'll start off fairly light and gradually pick up steam as labor progresses. Eventually the whole thing becomes quite gushy, gooey, and messy, and there will be a lot of underpad changing going on.

Some men can't stand the sight of blood and worry that they'll pass out during the delivery. If you're in that category, the good news is that it's uncommon for anyone to faint during delivery. Yes, it happens every once in a while, but not usually because of the blood. The majority of dads who *do* pass out do so because they've run out of fuel. So make sure you get plenty to eat and drink (and don't forget the breath mints). If you really have some issues with needles or the sight of blood, remember: You *never* need to be at the south end of the bed if you don't want to. There's plenty for you to do up north, at the head of the bed.

Once your baby is born, there will be even more blood. To start with, the placenta will need to separate from the wall of the uterus and be delivered. When that happens, you're likely to see a lot of blood—probably more than you've seen anywhere else but the movies. Most of that blood is coming from the placenta, and it's perfectly normal. Then, during the first few days after the delivery there will be even *more* blood. It's called *lochia* and may include occasional clots, which are basically uterine debris that's no longer needed since the pregnancy is over. Unless the chunks are bigger than tangerines, don't worry about it, it's normal. (The good news is that you aren't responsible for the clean-up.)

Keeping Her Hydrated and Fed

As you can imagine, losing all these fluids (not to mention perspiring and peeing all the time) can be dehydrating, so helping her replace them is an important part of your role. You'll also need to provide light food for her during early labor at home. Pretty much anything she feels like eating is fine, although most women in early labor won't be interested in anything heavy, like a steak or a calzone. Instead, go for something like a cup of soup, half a sandwich, toast, and so on. Encourage her to eat at least a little while in early labor—depending on how things progress, it could be a long time before her next meal.

As labor progresses—and especially after she's admitted to the hospital—your wife will most likely switch to clear liquids only: broth, tea, juice, Jell-O, and Popsicles, all of which are supplied by the hospital (make sure you scout out where the pantry is so you can have easy access to these). Hospitals generally insist on the clear-liquid regimen for several reasons. First, her stomach will no longer be busy digesting food because the blood is being diverted to the contracting uterus. And since she may end up tossing her cookies later, low or no solids isn't a bad idea anyway. As labor intensifies, her appetite will diminish and her need to replenish those depleted fluid reserves will increase. (After every couple of contractions, offer her a sip of clear liquids—it's a quick source of quick energy and is easily digestible.) Second, in the rare situation when a pregnant woman requires general anesthesia, the anesthesiologist will want her stomach as empty as possible due to the possibility of throwing up and then choking on the vomit.

The flip side of keeping hydrated is that you'll need to constantly remind her to empty her bladder—at least once every hour. (All the fluids combined with the baby's head sitting on her bladder makes the toilet a great place to labor.)

The McMoyler Maneuvers

As we talked about in Chapter 2, women's biggest fear about giving birth—and their biggest source of anxiety—is the pain. Over the course of my twenty-plus years as a labor and delivery nurse, I have helped many, many women deliver their babies with few medical interventions or none at all, and I have helped many others who had every possible high-tech intervention. For now, we're going to focus on low-intervention births. Labor and delivery nurses have seen it all and are not shy about giving you their assessment of how the labor is progressing; we know what works and what doesn't.

The most important thing to keep in mind is that in most cases, a bed is *not* the best place for a laboring woman to be. Once labor has started, most women will stay there—unless someone (you and your nurse) encourages her to make a change. In the following pages, I describe nine ways you can help get your wife out of bed and into different positions and environments that will help her cope with the pain and move labor along. I highly recommend that the two of you practice all of these McMoyler Maneuvers. That way, when labor begins, you'll both be familiar with the various options and how to do them. To be an effective support person on the day of labor, you'll need to get feedback about what's working and what's not. So start asking her; encourage her to tell you now and in the hospital.

Bad Dog

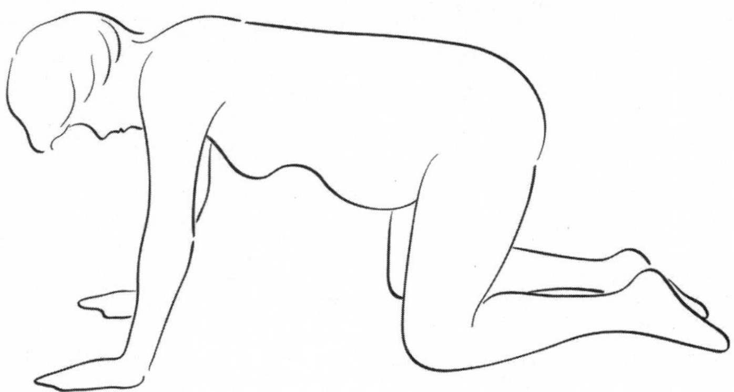

What it does

Simply being in a hands-and-knees position takes pressure off the low back and eases lower-back discomfort.

Bad Dog may also help the baby's head descend into the "desired," anterior position.

How to do it

1. Have her get on hands and knees with her back flat.
2. Tuck hips under as if someone were pulling a string from her belly button (just like a dog tucks its tail when scolded).
3. Her shoulders and upper back stay still, only the hips round under.
4. Make a slow, smooth motion to return to a flat back.
5. Breathe normally throughout.
6. Have her do thirty repetitions of this exercise every day. Better yet, do it together.
7. During labor, applying counterpressure with the heel of your hand to her lower back can really help.

Squatting

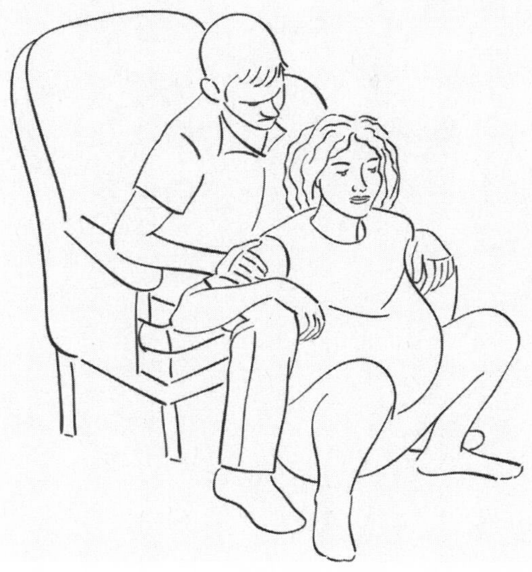

What it does

Her pelvis is built to give birth. This technique helps by opening the pelvis and allowing it to expand during labor.

Squatting also helps relax and stretch the muscles of the inner thighs, which will aid in pushing the baby out.

Squatting can be done out of the bed, upright, with hips in motion, and monitored if necessary, all at the same time.

How to do it

1. Have her squat down, knees far apart but right over the toes, or her heels can be under her buttocks.
2. You can sit in a chair behind her. She's squatting between your knees, facing out, and leaning back against you. Or, she can hold onto a couch, table top, the labor bed, or something else and simply come down into a squat. Some moms will prefer to be in a squat during the contraction, others in between contractions. Her decision. The point is to consider squatting during *labor* rather than waiting for the pushing stage.
3. Using the large quadriceps muscles in the thighs is a good idea, but don't overdue it, as these muscles will tire. So intersperse squatting with some of the other maneuvers.

Leaning over the Bed

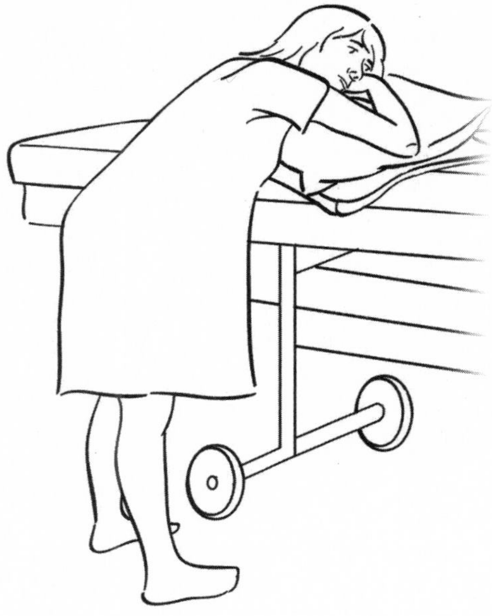

What it does

Utilizes gravity to take the pressure off her lower back, keep her pelvis in motion, and assist the baby in descending.

How to do it

1. Raise the hospital bed to the highest position and make a pile of pillows for her to lean over.
2. She stands facing the side of the bed, feet wide, knees relaxed, her upper body draped over the stack of pillows.
3. Her hips sway side to side.
4. If she wants, you can apply counterpressure to her lower back and/or get on the other side of the bed and in her face to help cope with pain.

Slow Dance

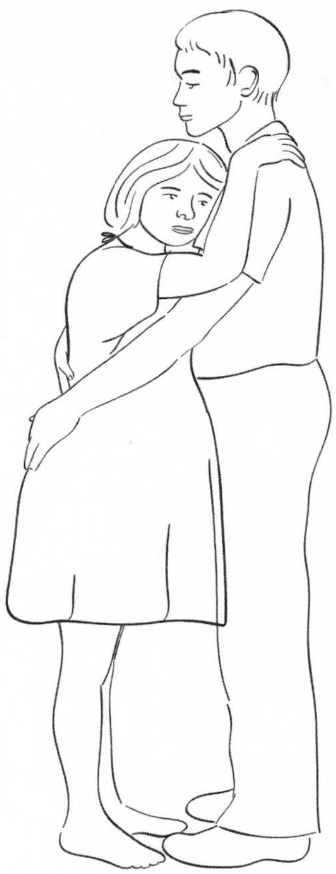

What it does

When she's in an upright position, contractions tend to be stronger, more regular, and more frequent.

How to do it

1. She puts her arms around your neck and hangs on you as if you were dancing at your junior prom.
2. Her feet should be shoulder-width apart, knees relaxed.
3. Her hips sway side to side.
4. This can be done anywhere: at the bedside, in the hallway, or in the shower.

Kneeling on the Bed

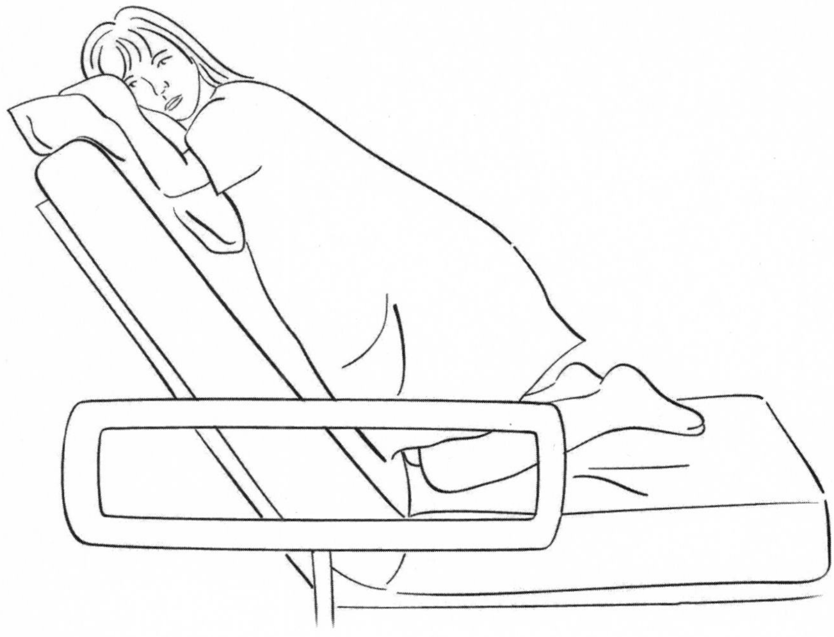

What it does

Allows for movement and gravity to do their work while her knees are cushioned by the mattress.

How to do it

1. Raise the head of the hospital bed to an upright position (the bed should now look like a letter L).
2. She kneels on the bed, facing the head of the bed.
3. She leans forward, arms across the head of the bed, supporting her upper body.
4. Getting into bed behind her will allow you to support her body, especially between contractions.

Rocking Chair

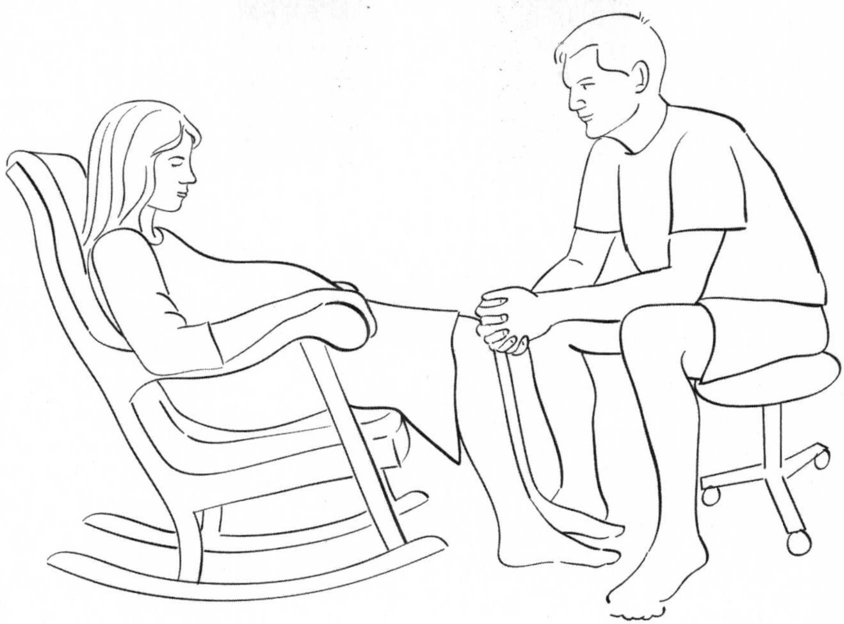

What it does

Helps her release and let go between contractions, which aids in coping. It may also enhance progress by allowing the baby to descend and/or making it easier to turn the baby into a better presentation.

How to do it

1. Put two pillows on a rocking chair: One goes under her butt, the other behind her back.
2. While she's seated in the rocker, you're on a low stool in front of her, mirroring for her during the peak and reminding her to release and let go in between contractions.

Toilet Trick

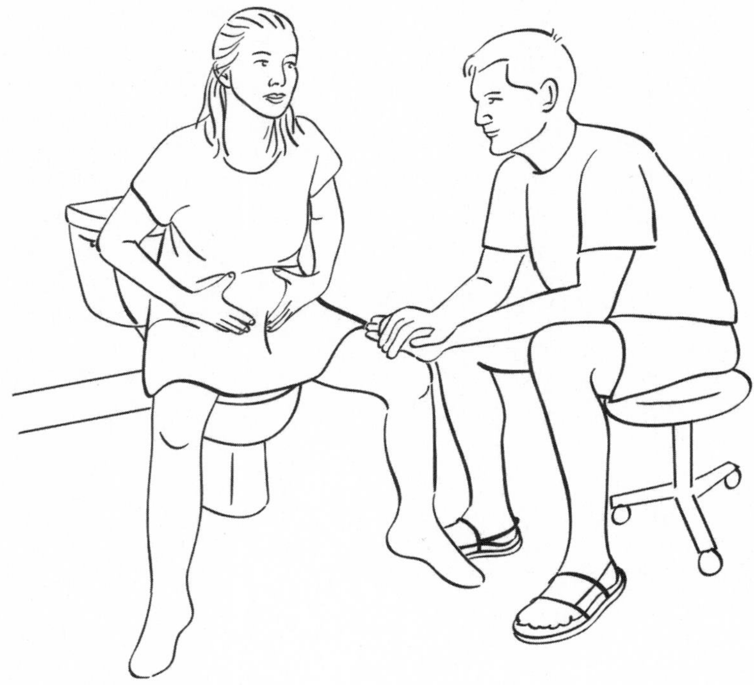

What it does

The toilet's hard seat activates pressure points in the buttocks that can help her cope with pain.

How to do it

1. In between contractions, help her into the bathroom and onto the toilet (a place where she may find it easier to relax).
2. Put a pillow behind her so she can lean back during the contractions.
3. Sit on a stool in front of her to do comforting or in-your-face mirroring.

Birth Ball

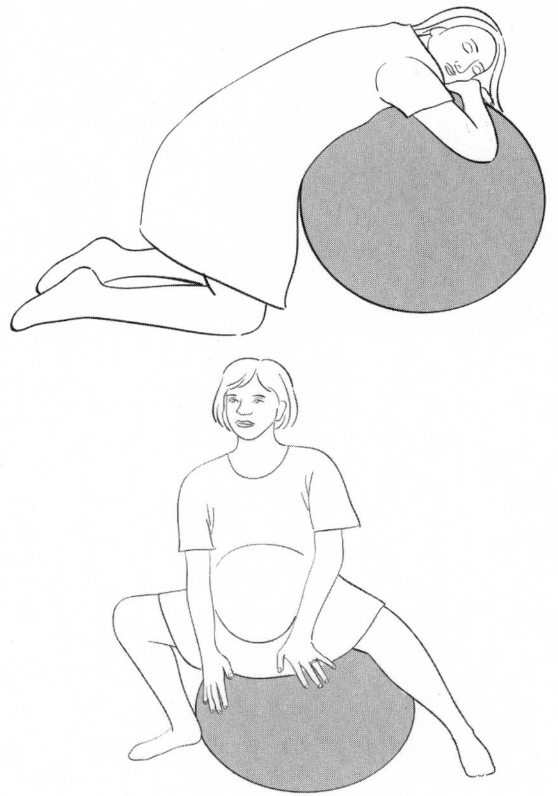

What it does

Sitting on a birth ball can enable her to involuntarily loosen her pelvic muscles. That will help her make labor more efficient.

How to do it

1. She can sit on the birth ball and slowly rock side to side and front to back. Leaning over the ball alleviates some pressure on the back and feels great.
2. Some hospitals have balls for you to use, others don't, so find out before you check in. You can find them at any sporting goods store.
3. Don't inflate the ball all the way. For labor, it's better if it's a little underinflated.

Shower Power

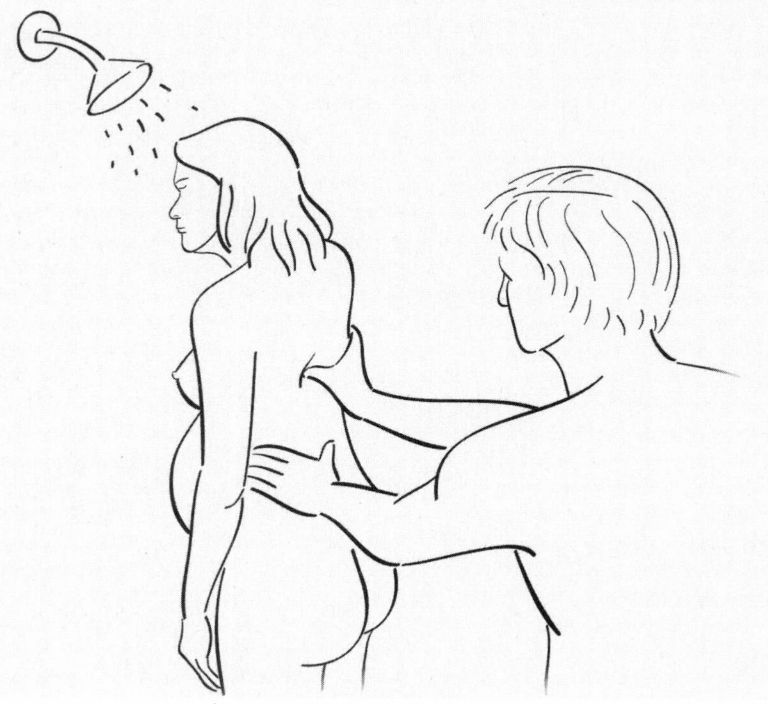

What it does

This is a McMoyler Method favorite and is the most effective noninvasive coping strategy. The sound and warmth of the water and the massage effect all enhance her ability to cope, which helps labor progress.

How to do it

1. With the water running, you can help her do as many of the other McMoyler Maneuvers as possible—slow dancing (or just leaning up against the wall), hands and knees, and Bad Dog are particularly good.
2. Over the course of the entire labor, she may take several showers, fifteen to forty-five minutes each.
3. There's a good chance you'll find yourself in the shower with her, or at least right outside, so don't forget to pack your swimsuit.
4. Get a bath blanket (actually a large flannel sheet that's stored in a warming unit).

> *If we hadn't learned the McMoyler Maneuvers, I don't know what I would have done. Leading up to my epidural, my husband and I must have slow danced for hours. As it turned out, this was my favorite position, and even though it left my husband's back stiff for a week, he never once complained. He was truly amazing throughout the entire process, never leaving my side and always there to center me.*
>
> —MARTINA L., NEW MOM

Given that you probably haven't done as much reading on pregnancy, labor, and delivery as your wife has, I'm including a very basic overview of the stages of labor and, more important, practical strategies (everything you *need* to know, instead of what's just nice to know).

Early Labor at Home

This is usually the longest phase—on average, about eight hours. Her contractions will come about seven to twenty minutes apart and will last about thirty seconds. At the very beginning of labor she'll be excited and probably eager for labor to get rolling. She may also be a little anxious and will want to keep you posted about every little detail. If you were to ask her, she'd tell you that the contractions "aren't all that bad"—kind of like a low backache or menstrual cramps. But over the course of this phase, her cervix will dilate (open up) from 0 centimeters to 3, and those contractions will gradually get stronger, longer, and closer together. She may also have diarrhea, which is the body's way of cleaning itself out.

Your Role in Early Labor

- You won't have to go to the hospital for at least a few more hours, so go out for your last meal alone and distract her—going to a movie or buying a little gift for her and the baby are always a hit.
- Keep her well-hydrated and bladder empty. Seems contradictory, but both are necessary.
- Record the frequency and duration of contractions. This will help more accurately gauge when it's time to head to the hospital. (You do not, however, need to record every contraction that occurs; every hour or so is fine. As they become more frequent, you will want to check more often.) Keep in mind that you will be asked about the pattern of contractions when you call to verify that it is indeed time to go.

Helping Her Cope

- When her contractions start to build in intensity and they become uncomfortable, you can help remind her to slow down her breathing and begin to focus. This is basically normal breathing, just slowed down a little, combined with focusing her eyes on a spot on the wall, a flower, a photo, or something else she finds calming and can concentrate on. At the same time, pay close attention to how she's reacting to her contractions. If she seems tense or is holding her breath, encourage her to release and let go, and be specific with your observations: drop shoulders, unclench teeth, breathe normally, and so on.

- At the beginning and end of every contraction, help her do a big inhale and a loud exhale, something like an exaggerated sigh.

Active Labor

This phase typically lasts around five hours, and you'll be in the hospital for most of it. Remember to call before you go—you want to be welcomed into Labor and Delivery with a room, a nurse, and your medical chart already pulled and ready to go. Labor and Delivery can get pretty busy, and they don't want people showing up on their doorstep unannounced. Once you are admitted, she'll be limited to drinking clear fluids. As her cervix dilates from 3 to 7 centimeters, there will be an increase in bloody show, which is normal. Contractions are now about five minutes apart and last about sixty seconds. They have higher peaks and are getting increasingly hard to cope with. During active labor, she won't be able to walk or talk during a contraction. She's very focused on herself and the work of labor. Her sense of humor is distinctly on hold, so if jokes tend to be your first line of defense, hold off. Nothing is going to seem funny to her right now.

Your Role in Active Labor

- Provide undivided attention, especially during contractions. Keep all of your communication clear and to the point.
- During contractions, get in her face and mirror for her what she needs to do to get through the peak. This includes any kind of vocalizing, *not* screaming. Help her keep the sounds low; a soft moaning sound is most helpful for this

kind of intensity. She should be moaning during each contraction and resting in between.

- You can increase her comfort in between contractions by offering sips of clear fluid, applying cold compresses, moistening her lips with lip balm, and fanning her.
- Between contractions, move in close to her and offer massages. Try her shoulder, or her hands or feet or scalp.
- Continually remind her that she's doing a fantastic job. She truly needs to hear this from you, so don't let the cat get your tongue.
- Make sure she empties her bladder at least every hour. Being upright on the way to and from the bathroom will help labor progress.

WHAT ARE YOU DOING IF SHE HAS AN EPIDURAL?

If your wife has an epidural, she won't need you to help her cope with the pain of the contractions. However, you can:

- Get some rest. Now that she's pain-free, pull out the hideaway bed (or cot) and lie down. Ask your nurse for pillows and blankets if you need them.
- Take a shower. Better do it now, because the next chance you have will likely be back at home after the baby is born.
- Grab a bite to eat. You can do this in the labor and delivery room if it doesn't disturb her. Otherwise, go to the hospital cafeteria or someplace nearby. Tell the nurse you're leaving and give her your cell number just in case.
- Make a few phone calls, outside of her room. Give your assigned phone-tree person the most recent updates.
- She will be lying on her side and will need to be turned to the other side once every hour. Be available to assist the nurse in turning her.
- Massage the side of her body that has been pressed into the sheets for the past hour. You'll actually see imprints of the hospital sheets on her skin. Rub them out using some lotion.

- Keep it quiet. She may not be feeling any pain, but she still needs to rest, so no TV or loud music.
- Remind her to let her body rest. If she isn't sleeping, encourage her to at least close her eyes. Dim the lights and put on some soft music. If she does go to sleep, tape a sign on the door saying, "Mom sleeping, please see the nurse."
- Suggest that she "see," in her mind's eye, her cervix opening to 10 centimeters, the baby descending downward, and herself pushing the baby into the world. This is what she gets to contribute now that she is epiduralized.

Helping Her Cope

- In-your-face mirroring
- Verbal anesthesia. "Great, terrific, open up even more, you're doing fine, stay with it, I'm right here with you . . ."
- Apply counterpressure. Ask her which helps more, high or low on the back, or closer to the tailbone.
- Get her up, walking, rocking, and changing positions. Do this only *between* contractions, not during.

> *My wife and I took a childbirth prep class at the hospital and we learned some breathing techniques I was supposed to get her to use during contractions. I guess I thought that they would be some kind of magic, that when we used those breaths (that we spent hours in class practicing) she would be able to deal with the pain. Well, we gave it our best shot, and the nurses were trying to help, but the breathing just wasn't working. The nurses ended up calling our doctor, who came in and recommended that my wife get an epidural. That turned out to be just the right decision. She went to sleep for a few hours, and when she woke up, they examined her and she was 10 centimeters. We couldn't believe it! A few hours later we were the proud parents of a baby boy.*

—ROBERT C., NEW DAD

THE PURRR TEST

Once every hour during labor, take a minute and give yourself this simple test to make sure you're doing everything you can to keep labor progressing. If you can answer yes to all of the following questions, you're doing fine. If there are any nos, you'll know what you need to do.

- Position. Every hour, is she up, walking, rocking, and changing positions?
- Urination. Every hour, is she emptying her bladder?
- Relaxation. Is she as relaxed as possible in between contractions? (Teeth unclenched, shoulders dropped, breathing slowly.)
- Rest. Is she releasing and letting go during those all-important minutes between contractions?
- Reassurance. Are you giving her verbal anesthesia in the form of encouragement?

FIGURING OUT WHERE YOU STAND WHEN SHE CAN'T

Throughout this chapter I've emphasized the importance of moving around during labor. But not every woman is going to be mobile. If your wife is, for whatever reason, laboring in bed, your place is at the *head* of the bed, right next to her face. The same goes for the actual delivery. You can't do any in-your-face mirroring, offer encouragement or reassurance, or much of anything if you're at the other end.

Transition

The good news is that this phase of labor is the shortest, only about an hour. The bad news is that it's also the most intense—her cervix will dilate from 7 to 10 centimeters—and that one hour can feel like an eternity. Contractions last for eighty to ninety seconds and are only two to three minutes apart (measuring from the beginning of one to the beginning of the next one), which makes them seem to come right on top of one another. She'll have increased bloody show, may feel the urge to bear down, and may become nauseated and/or vomit. Emotionally she's drained, and she may be crying from the fear and pain, and doubting whether she can actually make it the rest of the way.

Your Role in Transition

During transition, your nurse will be coming in more and more frequently to assess how your wife is coping. If your wife doesn't have an epidural, the nurse may actually stay with both of you the whole time. No matter how much preparation you've had, seeing your wife moving through incredibly intense contractions can be scary. If you get to a point where you feel like you're in over your head, help is only a push of a button away. Labor and delivery nurses aren't afraid of her pain. They know it's a sign of progress—the more intense it is, the sooner the pushing begins. Labor and delivery nurses all have their own bag of tricks, and they're extremely skilled at coming in during the steepest hurdle

---

WHOA, THAT WAS FAST . . . OR SLOOOOOW!

The time frames I'm giving in this chapter for each phase of labor are averages, which means that lots of people will experience it either faster or slower.

Second-timers usually have shorter labors, since the road was already paved by the first baby, although there will be first-timers who have what we call "precipitous labors," which go from early labor to transition, skipping active labor entirely. A labor like that may sound great, but there's a downside. Ask anyone who has been there and she'll tell you that labor was like a car with no brakes careening down a hill and she felt completely out of control. There's no time to regroup, just fasten your seat belt and hold on tight.

For first-time moms, fast-paced labors are the exception rather than the rule.

Overall, I'd rather have a first-time mom expect and prepare for the long haul and then be pleasantly surprised if labor moves along more efficiently.

---

to help guide her the rest of the way to 10 centimeters. Your nurse has seen it all a thousand times before and can make a big difference during a critical time.

Helping Her Cope

- Engage her mind. From the neck down, she's built to give birth, and her body knows what to do. What concerns me most is her mind, which is shouting, "I can't do this, I don't want to do this, I shouldn't be doing this, someone make this stop." By keeping her mind occupied—using visual, tactile, auditory approaches—you can help her get through those very intense contractions.
- Mirroring. At the beginning of each contraction, demonstrate a low, guttural moan. (Remember, talking to her won't get you very far; she needs to *see* what to do rather than hear about it.) As the contraction reaches the peak, move from moans to "heeeee" and "haaaaw" sounds, one long one for each exhale. Note: This is *not* the fast "whoo whoo whoo" or "he he he" that originate in the mouth or throat and are the staple of Lamaze. McMoyler Method "heeee haaaws" are deep and loud, and much closer to the natural human response to pain, which is decidedly *not* breathy. They move the pain up and out of the body.

> *The vocalizing techniques we learned saved us. My husband coached me through; we did the moans and the "heees" and the "haaaws," and when I went into the hysterical "I can't do this" wheezing, he was able to bring me back to center. We got into a rhythm—during the contractions he would remind me that we were on the down side and that the break was almost here. And once the contraction was*

> *over, he was great at getting me to release and let go. At one point I remember thinking that I was going crazy, and just in the nick of time, the nurse came in to back Sam up. He was hanging in there with me, but it was just too much. The nurse helped us get through a few more contractions, and it wasn't long before I was able to start pushing. It's true what they say: Pushing was not as painful as getting to 10 centimeters. I mean it, I pushed really hard, muscling down hard, and just did it.*
>
> —JENNA A., NEW MOM

- And more mirroring. Between contractions, help her release and let go by unclenching *your* fists and jaws, lowering *your* shoulders, and helping her whole body melt. The breaks will get shorter, and the more she can rest, the better she'll be able to cope with the next contraction.
- In-your-face verbal anesthesia. Lock eyes with her and tell her what a great job she's doing.
- Many women get the urge to push before they're completely dilated. If this is the case with your wife, your nurse will work with you to try to move your wife through that pushing urge. One excellent way to do this is to have her blow short puffs of air, as if she's blowing out a candle. This overrides her ability to bear down.
- Up, walk, rock, and change position. Some good choices for this phase are Shower Power, Slow Dance, and Bad Dog.

Pushing

You're almost there! At the end of these two hours, you'll finally get to meet the baby you've only imagined. Throughout this stage, your wife will get one-on-one nursing support. Even though your nurse now is in the room almost the entire time, you're still very much involved. Let me give you an example:

One time, I had just arrived in a patient's room at the beginning of my shift, and she was just about to start pushing. I looked around for her husband. He was sitting anxiously on the couch on the other side of the room. When I waved him over to join me at the bedside, he looked over each shoulder to see whom I could be talking to. I told him that we needed him to help, and he made his way slowly up and over to see what in the world he could possibly do. This dad-to-be was an enormous man and he ended up cradling his wife's upper body in his massive arms, supporting her head and neck with each push, and talked to her like his treasure in between contractions. When their baby boy was born, tears were streaming down his face as he cut the cord, amazed and surprised that he had actually helped his son be born.

Your Role in Pushing

- During pushing, your unconditional love and support are more important than at any other time. She has been through hours and hours of labor and now she's going to have to push like her life depends on it. She definitely doesn't want to be pushing for three or four hours (the average is two), and she wants to avoid "assistance" from vacuum extractors or forceps. To push effectively, she needs to bear down through the neck and chest, and use her abs to push down as if she was constipated. That's what propels babies downward. Fortunately, your nurse will be doing most of the directing at this point.
- Reassure her. The biggest worry women have while they're pushing is that if they push really hard they'll poop in the

bed. Well, it happens. A lot. Reassure her that if something comes out of the body ahead of the baby, it's only because she pushed so well that the baby's head has descended far into the birth canal.

- Even though pushing is hard physical work, what's happening in her head is just as important. She needs a second (and third and fourth) wind. Nurses are especially skilled at getting this job done. Let her hear your enthusiasm as you cheer her on.
- Ask your nurse to hold a warm compress on your wife's perineum. This is great for getting her to focus on exactly where to push (nurses frequently tell their patients to "push toward the warmth") and helps stretch the perineal tissues. The increased elasticity that results may help avoid an episiotomy.
- Update her. If you decide to hang out at the south end of the bed, tell her what's working when she pushes. Tell her when you see a little dark patch of wet baby head—this can be very motivating.
- Increase her ability to "coordinate" her efforts by having a mirror at the foot of the bed. Watching the baby begin to emerge can give her the motivation (and the strength that goes with it) to push more effectively.
- Follow the nurse's cues. She will be very good at customizing the pushing with different positions and telling your wife whether to hold her breath or exhale forcefully as she bears down.
- Count for her. It often helps during the push to count "one, two, three, four, five" to help her continue bearing down as long as she can with each push.

Helping Her Cope

- Using in-your-face mirroring, help her drop her shoulders, unclench her teeth, slow her breathing down, let her body melt into the bed in between pushes, and close her eyes, resting as much as she can until the next contraction comes. Some moms will actually nod off in between pushes.
- Hydrate her with sips of fluid or bites of ice. Put a cold washcloth on her forehead.
- Use verbal anesthesia, words of encouragement and praise. Cheer her on, love her, and remind her that the baby is almost here!

MomBox

There's nothing graceful or demure about pushing a baby out. In fact, it can be downright undignified. But who really cares? You're not there to audition, you're there to have a baby. So check your social graces at the door and give yourself permission to do whatever it takes to get to the goal.

Pushing with an Epidural

If she has an epidural, the feeling of "evacuation" has been removed—she's not going to get that overwhelming urge to bear down or push. Epidurals are often blamed for the lack of pushing ability, but we think that "pushing begins with attitude"—you bear down and put the pedal to the metal.

Here's what you can do to help:

- Help her conjure up the image of being constipated, and imagine how much better it would feel if she could just push this out of her body. (Moms who are pushing without an epidural feel the bowling ball moving through their body and get distinct cues to move it out.) The universal statement given to women in the second stage is, "Push like you need to move your bowels" (and, as mentioned above, poop does happen in labor).

- Most moms with epidurals will be directed to push holding their breath, no air or noise escaping. This is to create a sense of pressure below. If she's making noise and exhaling like a weight lifter, the push won't be as effective.
- Some nurses will want you to help hold her legs in "human stirrups" during the pushing. This is necessary because with the epidural she can't completely feel her legs or support them on her own.

If She Has a Cesarean

In Chapter 6, we discuss what will be happening immediately before, during, and after a cesarean, as well as what your role is throughout. Here are some of the highlights.

If your wife is having a scheduled cesarean, you'll be told the day and the time to arrive at the hospital. There'll be reams of paperwork to fill out and she'll be hooked up to a monitor that will track your baby's heartbeat. A nurse will take your wife's vital signs (temperature and blood pressure), and the anesthesiologist will drop by to walk you through the epidural procedure. Her OB or midwife will also stop by, just before the procedure.

At some point, you'll be taken outside the room while the nurses finish prepping her for the surgery. She'll be moved (by gurney, or in a wheelchair, or some women actually walk down the hall) to the operating room, where the anesthesiologist will do the epidural procedure. Meanwhile, you'll get some disposable scrubs of your own. Once your wife is all set, you'll be invited into the OR to take up your position on a stool near her head. Be prepared to see her now—she'll be sporting an oxygen mask or nasal prongs, her arms may be attached to arm boards (to keep them out of the sterile field), and there will be a drape across her body at about chest level. On the other side of that drape is where all the action will be happening.

> *Several weeks before the delivery, we discussed that if my wife had a cesarean, I would follow our child into the nursery while she was finishing up with the surgery. What a great decision. I had no idea how special it would be for me to spend that hour with our new little daughter. I helped the nurses wash her off, and I tried my first swaddle. I took a ton of pictures while we were still in the nursery. We were able to meet up with my wife in the recovery room in less than an hour, and then the nurse helped get the baby started breastfeeding almost immediately. I highly recommend that dads go to the nursery with their baby. It was a great time to bond. I also recommend that you talk in advance about where Dad is going to go.*
>
> —GEOFF H., NEW DAD

Your Role during a Cesarean

While you are both behind the sterile drape, waiting for the baby to be lifted into the world, you will definitely want to continue talking to her, offering reassurance; stay down close to her face and really stay present. There will be a lot going on around you, so aim for a little cocoon effect with her—it helps. Once your baby has been lifted out, you're on. A pediatrician will put your baby onto a nearby warming table. If you want to you can now move in that direction to snap a few photos and possibly cut the rest of the umbilical cord. The medical team will do a quick assessment of your baby, dry him off, clear the airway, attach a set of security bracelets that will match the ones you and your wife will both be given, and then get the baby swaddled. The nurse will carry the baby over to where Mom is (behind the drape) so that the three of you can spend a few minutes together before the baby goes off to the nursery.

The big decision at this point is whether you stay in the operating room with your wife or go with the baby to the nursery. I'm hoping that you'll have had this discussion before this moment. There is no right decision; it is completely up to the two of you and your individual needs and preferences.

> *Finally, I was escorted into the operating room for the surgery, and I was seated at the head of the operating table. I watched some of the surgery over the curtain, and it was surreal. I was talking to my wife and looking at this yellow belly as if it wasn't even a part of her (really interesting to watch the operation). The next thing I know, the doctor pulls out our baby, and I hear her first cry, and I get to inform my wife that we have a baby girl (we wanted to be surprised). I was absolutely beside myself with emotion, and I went over to the examination table (or whatever you call it) to help dry her off and cut the remaining cord . . . amazing.*
>
> —PAUL K., NEW DAD

CHAPTER

5

Whose Side Is the Medical Team On, Anyhow?

WHAT YOU'LL LEARN IN THIS CHAPTER:

- Your OB/midwife and labor and delivery nurses have your best interests in mind. Their goal is to guide you through a safe and healthy delivery.
- Innovation and technology are there to assist labor and save lives—*not* to complicate matters, as some would have you believe.
- How to overcome the fears or concerns you may have about hospitals and medical staff.

IMAGINE FOR A moment that you or someone in your family needs a root canal, or a broken bone set, or heart bypass surgery. Chances are, you'll spend some time getting recommendations and trying to find the best facility and the best people to do the job. It probably wouldn't occur to you to question the dentist's or orthopedist's or cardiologist's motives or loyalties or to wonder whether they really have your best interests at heart. You'd trust the medical (and dental) professionals to do their job, and "whose side are they on?" is a question that wouldn't even cross your mind.

If that's true—and I think for most people it is—why doesn't the same logic apply to obstetricians and labor and delivery nurses? Why are so many people suspicious of their motives, and why are they so often seen as the enemy?

To a large extent, the answer has to do with politics and patient education, two things that often go hand in hand. Traditional childbirth prep methods—in particular Bradley and Lamaze—tend to look at the medical team as agenda-driven procedure-pushers who are often more concerned with their own convenience than the needs of their patients.

McMoyler Method, on the other hand, has a completely different view. We believe that while there are occasional bad apples, the overwhelming majority of doctors, nurses, and other health care professionals are your allies, fully committed to providing you the best emotional and physical care. They have years of experience delivering babies, and when they recommend medications or procedures, it's because they genuinely think it's the best thing for you and your baby in the given situation.

Am I suggesting that doctors and nurses can do no wrong and that you blindly obey everything they say? Absolutely not. I *am* suggesting, though, that you invest some time learning everything you can about what's *probably* going to happen during labor and delivery, and what *might* happen (you've already taken a giant step in that direction by reading this book). I'm also suggesting that you get recommendations and find the best doctor and the best hospital for *you.* (I understand that, depending on your insurance coverage, you may not have as many choices as you'd like, but in almost every case you'll have at least *some* options.) Once you're satisfied with the OB or midwife you've decided on and the hospital you've chosen, trust them to do their job—at least as much as you'd trust your dentist to do a root canal. Despite what you see on television, obstetrical emergencies are rare, so the chances are very good that you'll have a relatively uneventful delivery—and that you'll never have to deal with a "what if" scenario.

Starting the day you and your husband commit to having a baby—and continuing throughout the pregnancy—your head will be filled with questions and concerns: Can we afford this? Have we completely lost our minds? How much will it hurt? Will I be able to handle the pain? How long will it last? Will my husband be there for me? Will we be good parents? And on and on. The *last* thing you need to add to that jumble of worries is whether the medical team is going to be pushing you in directions you don't want to go, or to do things you don't want to do. Those are legitimate concerns, which in many instances can be alleviated (or at least minimized) ahead of time, so that when the day comes to deliver the baby, you're comfortable with your decisions and can focus on the task at hand.

I'm sure that you've been hearing all sorts of stories—positive and negative—about birth and people's experiences with doctors, nurses, and hospitals. And I can guarantee that you'll hear plenty more before your baby comes. My goal in this chapter is to tell you what I know to be true, based on my experiences working in a number of hospitals during my twenty-plus years as a labor and delivery nurse, as well as what I've heard from dozens of my colleagues.

Although it may sound as though McMoyler Method and traditional childbirth methods are at opposite ends of the scale, McMoyler Method is actually pretty much in the middle. Back in 1900, almost all babies were born at home, and childbirth was women's work, in the true sense of the phrase: Laboring mothers were generally surrounded by other women, some of whom had training as midwives; others didn't. But as families started leaving the family farm and moving to smaller homes in the city, home births became less practical. So mothers began to give birth in hospitals, and doctors began taking over. In 1935, half of all babies were born in hospitals; by 1970, it was over 95 percent.

Here's where Bradley and Lamaze come in. They started wondering whether the pendulum had swung too far, and whether doctors and hospitals were getting *too* involved. And they were right. In their well-intentioned attempts to avoid infections, doctors turned childbirth into a sterile, medical process—and not always a particularly nice one. Many doctors were arrogant, so concerned about the clinical side of the equation that they often forgot about the human part. There are plenty of stories of women who had to have their pubic hair shaved and had their legs in stirrups for hours at a time, all in the name of maintaining the "sterile field." And *everyone* had an episiotomy, no questions asked.

Doctors started relying heavily on forceps to accomplish deliveries. Women were instructed to labor flat on their backs in bed and were routinely given "twilight sleep," a cocktail of drugs that knocked them out and erased their memory of the birth. Narcotics and spinals became increasingly popular, and most babies were born in stark operating rooms (with no dads allowed). The cesarean birth rate rose like a rocket, from 4.5 percent in 1965 to over 22 percent just two decades later. Today it's close to 30 percent. (We'll talk more about cesareans later in the chapter.) As much as I hate to admit it, the truth is that some doctors probably *did* schedule cesareans for convenience rather than the best interests of the patient.

The Bradley and Lamaze movements deserve credit for getting the pendulum to start swinging in the other direction. However, in the process, they created something of a backlash. Couples started demanding fewer interventions and more control over their birth experience, in other words, a more "normal" childbirth. Unfortunately, the whole "normal" birth attitude went too far, and couples became overly wary of doctors and nurses and our supposedly hidden agendas. Women started getting the message that if they didn't feel every last ripple of pain—no matter how hard or for how long—they'd failed as women and as mothers. (We'll talk more about the impact of these feelings of failure in Chapter 7.)

And that brings us back to McMoyler Method, which occupies the space between the two extremes: (a) an unmedicated, intervention-free birth where doctors are hardly involved and (b) giving birth, while unconscious, in a cold, sterile, antiseptic hospital room. As we see it, the medical team is there to help you bring your baby into the world in the safest, most efficient way possible. End of story. If you want a low-to-no-intervention birth, they'll support you any way they can. But if something happens that jeopardizes your or your baby's health, they'll do whatever is necessary.

> *What's my role in labor and delivery? Primarily, it's to support the laboring mom and provide as much support and guidance as I can. Even under the best of circumstances, giving birth isn't a particularly enjoyable experience. To start with, I pay very close attention to the way Mom looks and behaves and try to give her the kind of help she needs—for every patient it's a little different. I try to keep my patients out of bed as much as possible, and I'll encourage Mom and her partner to try different positions, like using a birthing ball or getting into the shower. I really believe that what I do can have a big impact. As a nurse, I work hard to facilitate the birth process, keeping the doctors apprised of the patient's situation, maintaining the health of Mom and Baby, and providing support and suggestions along the way. Getting a mom through a particularly tough spot in labor and making sure she knows what her options are can sometimes make the difference between a vaginal birth and a cesarean.*

—JANICE, LABOR AND DELIVERY NURSE

MEDICAL TECHNOLOGY—SAVING LIVES

In 1900, 100 babies out of every 1,000 died before their first birthday. And 10 of those 1,000 mothers died giving birth or of pregnancy-related problems. Today the infant mortality rate is less than 10 per 1,000, and the maternal mortality rate is 12 to 13 per *100*,000. That's a 90 percent drop in infant mortality and a 99 percent drop in maternal mortality. Personally, I've seen many close calls that were averted thanks to the availability of medical technology.

IN THE TRENCHES

As a way of illustrating what a labor and delivery nurse does, let me tell you about an actual experience I had with a patient. Almost every nurse I've ever met has done similar things with her patients.

I had just come on shift, and the nurse who was getting off was briefing me on the patients. One in particular had an epidural and was getting pretty good pain relief, with the exception of a "window" on her uterus that wouldn't numb completely. Emotionally, she was starting to lose it. She had been pushing for over an hour and her focus was waning, her energy was slipping, and we knew that if this kept up, she could be heading for the operating room. When I entered the room, I found the dad sitting in a chair, staring out the window, and the laboring woman's mother sitting in another chair wringing her hands. The patient was breathing rapidly, her brow was knitted, her hands and teeth were clenched—and this was in *between* contractions. I introduced myself and told her that I was going to try to help her with the pushing. She gripped me and said that she desperately wanted to avoid a cesarean. I asked the dad and grandma to come over to the bedside, and I assigned each of them a leg to hold in "human stirrups" while I talked Mom through the contractions, helping her push like her life depended on it. In between contractions, I modeled for Dad how to get in close to her and tell her she was doing great, and to use his own body language to demonstrate for her how to unclench her fists and release the tension. I got Grandma to chime in with supportive words like "We love you, honey. Let's have this baby!" The four of us got into a nice rhythm of serious pushing, resting as completely as possible, and being loved and nurtured in between pushes. After less than an hour of this, the baby was born vaginally. Mom practically floated over to the postpartum unit, so elated to have avoided what had seemed like an inevitable cesarean.

Unfortunately, many traditional childbirth prep instructors (most of whom have little or no medical training of their own) teach content that simply isn't realistic. They continue to educate—actually, "indoctrinate" is a better word—their students that the medical community's motivations are suspect and that expectant couples need to protect themselves against unwanted and unnecessary interventions.

Ordinarily, I wouldn't waste time arguing these points, but since they've been the cornerstones of traditional childbirth education for so many years, it's time to set the record straight. I want you to hear their version of the story—which is too often based on politics and conjecture. Then I'll give you a realistic picture from the McMoyler Method viewpoint, which is based on the latest scientific research and literally thousands of labor and delivery experiences.

They say: Home births are as safe as or safer than hospital births.

The truth: As a rule, only women who know they're low-risk would even consider having a home birth, while anyone who has been told by her doctor that she's high-risk will opt for the hospital route. Given that hospitals are handling all the high-risk patients, it's no wonder that they have a higher rate of emergency procedures and birth-related problems than home births do. Does that mean that if you're a low-risk expectant mom it's okay to have your baby at home? Yes, but I would advise against it. There's no question that a home birth offers a more familiar environment and a friendly, warm ambience (it is *home,* after all). I know many women who have delivered their babies at home (and we're still friends) and I know it can be a wonderful and powerful experience. By and large, a low-risk woman giving birth at home will be fine (although many women who *intend* to give birth at home end up going to the hospital because they need pain-management options or because their midwife is concerned about the baby's heart rate). The big question remains: What if something were to happen and you needed emergency medical care? Sometimes even being next door to the hospital is too far away. I know that you want to do everything possible to minimize the potential harm to yourself and your baby, so why take any risks at all—particularly when they're completely avoidable?

> *When I look back at the patients I've nearly lost, the number-one reason was an unanticipated postpartum hemorrhage, usually caused by an amniotic fluid embolism. I was unable to predict a single one of those massive hemorrhages. When one happens, patients need blood clotting factors now and being even a few minutes away from the hospital is a few minutes too far.*
>
> —LAURIE G., OB/GYN

> *Throughout the pregnancy I was considered very low-risk and since neither my husband nor I wanted any medical interventions, we were seriously considering a home birth. But our OB recommended against it and I'm so glad he did. After about twenty-seven hours of labor, the baby's heartbeat dropped through the floor and I had an emergency cesarean. They discovered that she had the cord wrapped around her neck three times. If we hadn't had a skilled medical team right there, who knows what would have happened?*
>
> —ELIZABETH R., NEW MOM

They say: Hospital medical teams don't support "normal" (unmedicated) childbirth.

The truth: Most hospitals—and McMoyler Method—firmly support unmedicated, low-intervention childbirth, as long as that's what the mother wants, her labor is progressing, and she and the baby are both tolerating the labor process well. If you want a natural birth (meaning avoiding interventions and medication), your doctors and nurses will do everything they can to move you along in that direction. But if all of the noninvasive, nonmedical options haven't adequately helped labor progress or increased your ability to cope with contractions, they'll definitely want to introduce medical options. The point is to stay focused on having your baby. It's not a contest, and you don't get points for what you do or don't do during labor. It's all about making choices and decisions along the way. Once your healthy baby is in your arms, all the pressure to give birth a certain way will go up in a puff of smoke.

> *As a labor and delivery nurse, my goal is to help you have your baby in the safest, most memorable way possible. And I'll support you in having the kind of birth you want to have. What you have to understand is that childbirth is extremely unpredictable and things can change suddenly. I've got twelve years of experience delivering babies and if something happens that puts you or your baby at risk, I'm going to do everything possible to keep people alive and healthy. That may mean that your birth experience might be different than you imagined it would be, but at the end of the day, isn't the real goal to have a healthy baby?*
>
> —LAURA R., LABOR AND DELIVERY NURSE

They say: Standard labor-management techniques such as intravenous (IV) fluids and intermittent fetal heart rate monitoring are invasive and unnecessary, and interrupt mobility.

The truth: 80 percent to 90 percent of laboring women get IV fluids at some point during labor, and about the same percentage have electronic fetal monitoring. Sounds like a lot, but whether those procedures are actually unnecessary is debatable. Medical professionals are trained to try to reduce risk. Instead of waiting for problems to arise and then reacting, they may opt for taking a step designed to help the patient *avoid* the problem before it happens.

It's extremely easy to get dehydrated over the course of hours and hours of laboring. IV fluids provide a much bigger drink than anything you could possibly consume by mouth. Babies typically respond very positively to IV fluids, in terms of heart rate and levels of movement and activity. We suggest talking to your nurses about having your IV line "capped" until/unless you actually need it.

Electronic fetal monitors are extremely useful tools. They're typically used intermittently (roughly once every hour during labor) and allow the medical team to see how well the baby is tolerating the labor and delivery. Without them, we would have absolutely no way of telling how the baby is really doing. Dr. Julian Parer, nationally recognized perinatologist at the University of California, San Francisco, puts it this way: "With each contraction, it is as if the baby is diving down to touch the drain in the deep end of a swimming pool. It catches a big breath as it dives downward, touches the drain, waits at the bottom of the pool for the peak of the contraction to be over, and then pushes off the bottom to pop through the water and catch a breath." As kids, we all had similar kinds of swimming pool experiences, and it was fine (and fun) because we did it only once or twice. But unborn babies have to dive down to the bottom of the pool with every contraction, over and over for hours and hours. Sometimes they get exhausted. When that happens, it's time for technology to step in.

Many people believe that being monitored requires staying in bed with the covers up. Not true. In fact, you can do most of the

McMoyler Maneuvers while you're being monitored. The leads or cables that the monitors are attached to allow you to walk all the way around the bed, sit in the rocking chair, lean over the bed, sit on the birth ball, slow dance, and pretty much everything except get in the shower. So if you're being monitored and you want to get up, in most cases all you have to do is ask. (If you're giving birth in a hospital where they use wireless telemetry monitors, you'll be able to walk from one end of the building to the other!)

> *A hospital is a hospital, and almost by definition there's not a whole lot there that's "natural." When an expectant couple shows up here, they need to know that we have legal and ethical obligations to take the best care of them possible. And while that doesn't always include an epidural and IV, it almost always involves some electronic monitoring of Mom and Baby.*
>
> —ARLENE L., LABOR AND DELIVERY NURSE

They say: Having an epidural leads to all sorts of other unnecessary interventions.

The truth: Having an epidural does trigger a whole cascade of other interventions, including IV fluids, a catheter in the bladder, and sometimes Pitocin. (We talk about this in much more detail in the next chapter.) Are those interventions truly necessary? The answer is simple: yes. For example, if you have an epidural, you probably won't be able to get up to go to the toilet; a catheter takes care of that problem. Epidurals can sometimes spread out contractions and slow down labor; Pitocin helps keep those contractions coming and labor progressing. The big question is whether those interventions are dangerous. And the answer is that there's no strong scientific evidence that indicates that they are.

It's all about knowledge and preparation. If you've done your homework and you know what to expect, you're not going to feel as if you were blindsided by a bunch of unexpected procedures.

They say: Hospitals intervene in "normal" births and do cesareans even when there's no medically sound reason for doing so, for one or both of the following reasons: (a) there are financial incentives and (b) it's more convenient for the doctors.

The truth: This is absurd. For a vaginal birth, there'll usually be one OB and one nurse in the room. For a cesarean, there are at least twice that number. Most insurance companies reimburse the same amount regardless of whether the birth is vaginal or by cesarean. Cesarean section patients stay in the hospital twice as long (four days versus two for a vaginal delivery) and require more postpartum recovery (four to six weeks versus two to three for vaginal). All in all, OBs collect about the same amount per hour either way. But you don't have to take my word for it. By law, women are entitled to full informed consent before making any decision about medical procedures or surgery. According to a recent national study, 90 percent of mothers said they didn't feel pressured to have any intervention. And only 2 percent thought there was no medical reason for their cesarean.

> *As anesthesiologists, our job is to relieve pain. And we are, I must say, pretty popular in labor and delivery. We don't push medications or epidurals on women in labor. We do, however, think that epidurals are certainly a great option for women who want them. Medical science and technology continue to make great strides in what, when, and how we administer pain medication. If I were a woman giving birth, I'd absolutely choose to have an epidural—it looks like it hurts like hell!*

—MARTIN W., ANESTHESIOLOGIST

Cesareans: How Many Is Too Many?

Cesarean section is the most common surgery for women of childbearing age in the United States, and nearly 30 percent of pregnant women give birth that way. Critics say that's too high, but there's no agreement on what "too high" means and what an "ideal" rate might be. (This debate has been the subject of a number of books and is beyond the scope of what we can get into here. Suffice it to say that both sides make valid points. If you're interested in learning more, I've included several resources on page 246.)

One thing almost everyone *does* agree on is that a cesarean should be done only when absolutely necessary. And like any other major surgery, cesareans can pose risks to Mom and Baby—risks any responsible health care professional would try to minimize. For example, babies delivered by cesarean tend to be born with more fluid in their airways (which would have been squeezed out in a vaginal birth). Cesarean-section moms have a higher risk of infection and a longer recovery, and they may have a little more trouble conceiving again and a higher risk of uterine rupture in future pregnancies.

Without taking sides, let me take you through some of the factors that may contribute to the increase in the cesarean rate.

- **Convenience versus liability.** As I mentioned above, I disagree with the idea that OBs are performing cesareans for their own convenience. There may have been some isolated incidences of this happening a few decades ago, but it's simply not going on today. In some cases, what looks like doctor convenience is actually fear of liability. If a situation comes up during labor where there's some risk to the mom or the baby, some OBs will recommend an immediate cesarean. That may not be what they'd like to do, but the sad reality is that they're afraid they'll be sued if they don't. If something were to go wrong, everyone would demand to know how come the medical team hadn't done everything possible to reduce the risk. It's unfortunate that often doing a cesarean is what lawyers and insurance companies consider "reducing risk." I should add, though, that not all OBs fall into this camp.

> *I don't think I ever think about lawsuits or malpractice when I do an emergency cesarean because of a problem with the baby. In many other branches of medicine we usually have second chances—another surgery, a new drug, an alternative treatment, etc. But in obstetrics there are no second chances. Taking a risk during labor could have an effect that lasts from birth all the way through the eighty-year life expectancy of that child. And the entire family—siblings, parents, grandparents—will be affected as well. As far as I'm concerned, if just one baby retains IQ points or motor abilities that might have been otherwise lost, the trade-off is probably worthwhile.*
>
> –JASON A., OB

- **Previous cesarean.** Women who've had one cesarean have about a 70 percent chance of having another one with their next pregnancy. This is in part due to the weakening of the uterine muscle that occurred with the first cesarean. In subsequent pregnancies, the constant contractions for hours and hours may be too much to ask of the uterus, putting it at risk for rupturing. The decision to attempt a VBAC (vaginal birth after cesarean) is made on a case-by-case basis. If you're considering one, bring up the issue at your next OB visit.

Your doctor will look back at your previous pregnancy, review why the first cesarean was done and where on the uterus the original incision was made, and make an informed recommendation about the safest route for you to deliver.

- **Mom's age.** The cesarean rate for women under twenty is about 16 percent; for women over forty, it's almost 50 percent. This is in part due to the fact that the uterus is a muscle, and like any other muscle, its strength decreases with age. A woman whose uterus struggles to force a baby out when she's forty-two might very well have been able to deliver the same size baby with no problem when she was twenty-two.

DadBox

If you're a sports fan, you've probably noticed that athletes start losing some of their spring as they get older, usually in their mid- to late thirties. The same goes for your wife's uterus, which is in for a long, intense game on the day your baby will be born. As your wife ages, her uterus—which is a muscle—simply isn't going to perform as well. All else being equal, a woman in her forties will have a much harder time pushing a baby through her pelvis than a woman in her twenties. Her contractions may slow down or stop altogether, necessitating labor augmentation with Pitocin. Sometimes, though, even Pitocin can't get a stalled labor back on track and a cesarean may be required.

- **Twins, triplets, technology, and more . . .** Because fertility declines with age, many women in their thirties and forties need a little high-tech assistance to get pregnant. Many of these technologically supported pregnancies result in two or more fetuses, which may automatically put the mother into the high-risk category. (The same is true for the increasing number of younger women who have fertility treatments.) Besides carrying multiples, older moms also have to contend with the issue of uterine strength, as mentioned above. Scheduling cesareans for multiple births is getting more and more common because doing so allows the hospital to make sure the right medical team is available, book the operating room and a postpartum bed, and prepare the nursery for multiples, all of which increase the odds of a good outcome. The decision to schedule a cesarean for twins has a lot to do with the position of the babies. If both are head down (a situation called *vertex/vertex*), vaginal birth is often recommended. However, if either baby is not head down, cesarean is usually the delivery option of choice, at least for one of them. The two of you should discuss the pros and cons of both vaginal and cesarean births so you can make the most informed choice.

- **Obesity.** In case you were out of the country for the past few years, we're in the middle of an obesity epidemic. Obese women are at risk for all sorts of pregnancy complications (including hypertension, diabetes, and blood clots) that put them into the high-risk category.
- **Maternal choice.** As more and more celebrity moms are scheduling their cesareans, noncelebrity women are following suit. The primary reason for these elective cesareans is control. For some women, being able to predetermine the date and time their baby will be born is huge. An expectant mom can work right up to the last minute or can make sure to have the baby at a particularly convenient time for herself or her family. (If you're in the avoiding-pain category, consider the trade-off: several hours of pain—most of which can be eliminated with an epidural—versus up to six weeks of not being able to go up and down the stairs, stand up straight without hurting, or drive a car.)

> *I was definitely planning to have an unmedicated birth, but after seventeen hours of labor, I was only 2 centimeters dilated and was exhausted and in agony. At that point, our nurse asked whether I would consider an epidural, and I could hear my instructor's voice in my head, warning me that the hospital staff would try to push all sorts of unnecessary drugs and procedures on us. So I just about bit the nurse's head off and refused. After three more hours and no more progress, she gently tried again, and that time I went for it. And, boy, am I glad I did. I'm still irritated that I waited for so long, for no apparent reason, and regret some of the ideas I came in with, like the nursing staff is the enemy—it was obvious that they were doing everything they could to help me with the pain. I apologized to that nurse later.*
>
> —EMMA P., NEW MOM

Conversation Starters

When arriving at the hospital, most couples bring along a change of clothes, some toiletries, and perhaps a few other items. Many of them also arrive with a lot of *psychological* baggage—fears, thoughts, worries, concerns, and memories about hospitals and the people who work there. It's essential that you and your husband leave that baggage outside the hospital door. You're about to have a completely unique experience and you need to go into it with as few preconceived notions as possible. The questions below are designed to help the two of you accomplish that goal.

- How do both of you feel about hospitals and medical staff?
- Have either of you or anyone you know had any negative experiences with hospitals? How about with the specific hospital where you're delivering? (Going into the same hospital where

a relative died, or where you were taken with a childhood trauma, can easily bring up all sorts of fears and worries.)

- Have you read, heard, or seen anything that has specifically caused you to feel worried or afraid? This would include books or articles on pregnancy and childbirth, or images from a television show or movies.
- Have you discussed your concerns with your doctor? He or she will be able to answer all your questions and, hopefully, put your mind at ease.
- Once you've talked about all of this, can you put your fears aside? If after having these conversations with your husband and discussing any concerns with your OB, you're still scared, let your doctor know. You may benefit from some other form of short-term, focused therapy, or another alternative that your OB can recommend.

In my years as a labor and delivery nurse, I've seen hundreds of Bradley and Lamaze students come to the hospital suspicious of me and the rest of the hospital staff. Every labor and delivery nurse I've ever worked with can say the same. You and your husband are going to be spending several days working closely with a group of highly trained people who deliver babies for a living. As you can probably imagine, hostility toward the medical staff is no way to start what is going to be a pretty intimate relationship. In the next chapter, we'll talk about the specific role each member of the medical team plays in caring for you and your baby, as well as how you and your partner can forge strong relationships with the doctors and nurses who will be doing everything they can to make sure you leave the hospital with exactly what you came there to get.

CHAPTER

6

Who Are These People? Introducing the Medical Team and How to Have the Best Relationship with Them

WHAT YOU'LL LEARN IN THIS CHAPTER:

- Who all the members of the medical team are, and what each one of them does
- The vocabulary of labor and delivery; an overview of the most common words, procedures, and concepts that may come up during the birth process
- Tried-and-true strategies for creating close, trusting, working relationships with the hospital medical staff

A Whole New Kind of Relationship

If you think about it for a few minutes you'll probably agree that the relationship you're going to have with your medical team is quite a bit different from most other relationships. To start with, you're about to spend at least two days with a group of people you hardly know, who will repeatedly poke and prod every possible orifice, and who will be getting to know you and your husband during what is likely to be the most stressful time of your lives. And then you leave. Doesn't sound like the makings of a strong bond, does it? But it really needs to be. The truth is that the better your working relationship with the medical team, the better your childbirth experience will be.

For much of the time after you check into the hospital, everything seems to be moving slowly (it'll seem *incredibly* slow). As you get closer to the actual birth, it's going to feel like Grand Central Station. Things will speed up, people and supplies will be coming in and out of the room, they'll start tossing around all sorts of strange words and acronyms. It'll be a big blur—albeit an important one. If you're going to have the kind of birth experience you want and if you're going to feel that you have some say in what's going on, it's essential that you and your partner familiarize yourselves with as much of what's happening around you (and *to* you) as possible. Let's start with who may come into the room, in order of appearance.

- **Labor and delivery nurse.** The first thing to know about labor and delivery nurses is that they generally love what they do. It takes a special individual to work in a fast-paced, emotionally charged environment; provide ongoing care for you, your baby, and perhaps one more patient; keep you, your husband, and your OB/midwife informed about how labor is going; explain your options and make recommendations for ways to help labor progress; engage with the family (husband, parents, in-laws, siblings, and others); provide emotional support and ensure that your needs are being met; stay cool, calm, and collected (not to mention pleasant, honest, and direct); stay at your bedside during labor and pushing; and then come back the next day to do it all over again. Whew! That's an awful lot of hats to wear.

As far as education, a labor and delivery nurse may have a two-year associate's degree in nursing, a four-year degree in nursing, or even a master's degree. Regardless of her education, she (sometimes he) will have taken specialized courses covering labor, delivery, fetal monitoring, and newborn care.

In the event that you're delivering by cesarean, your labor and delivery nurse most likely will go with you and become the circulating nurse, getting you situated, helping the operating-room team set up for surgery, getting Dad seated behind the drape, helping you and your husband hold the baby for a few minutes after the delivery, and ultimately taking the baby to the nursery for an in-depth assessment.

OH, NURSE, WE HARDLY KNEW YE

Since the average labor lasts eight to twenty-four hours and the average nursing shift is only eight to twelve hours, there's a good chance that you'll see more than one nurse before your baby is even born. Couples often worry that when their first nurse leaves for the day, they'll have to re-establish the working relationship with a completely new one. The worry is understandable, but most of the time this kind of scenario works out in your favor. First, you're getting a fresh, energized nurse. Second, your previous nurse will have given her replacement a complete, detailed report on your labor thus far. You'll still want to introduce yourselves and fill in the new nurse on your labor-and-delivery wish list. All she wants to know is that you have reasonable expectations and that you're prepared to be flexible if the need arises.

- **Midwife.** There are two types of midwives, both of which provide support during labor and delivery and ultimately deliver babies born vaginally. Certified midwives (CM) have been through specialized training programs in childbirth (which may include an internship with a physician and/or other midwife). CMs aren't recognized by every state, and many insurance companies won't pay for them. Much more common (and more widely recognized) are certified nurse-midwives (CNM). They are registered nurses who have also completed a specialized midwifery training program. A CNM who has hospital privileges can function independently within a hospital setting. However, it's rare to find one who practices on her own—most are part of an established obstetric practice. The reason for this is that in the event that a pregnancy or labor becomes a high-risk situation, a midwife's skill set is somewhat limited when compared to a physician's. Midwives are known for providing in-depth prenatal care and being invested in avoiding interventions when possible.

- **Your physician.** Unless you've chosen to have your family practitioner do the delivery (which is uncommon), we're talking about your OB/GYN. He or she will be in a few times while you're in labor to check on your progress, assess the baby's heart rate, help make decisions, and generally see how you're doing. Most of the labor management will happen from afar, via phone updates from your nurse. When you get to the pushing stage, your OB will arrive to handle the delivery.
- **The OB on call** (sometimes called the "doc in the box"). On-call doctors stay in the labor and delivery unit for eight to twelve hours. They eat and sleep there, assess patients, are available to answer questions, will assist during a cesarean, handle "emergent moments" (meaning that something unexpected happens that requires a fast response), and will deliver your baby if your own doctor can't be there.

Many expectant women worry about having someone other than their regular OB caring for them. I understand completely, and I clearly remember feeling that way myself when we were expecting our first baby. Even though I knew that it wasn't entirely reasonable, I really hoped that my OB would be there that day. She wasn't.

You've probably spent months, if not years, building your relationship with your OB. But the reality is that they can't possibly be available for every single patient day and night. They're seeing other patients in their office, delivering babies, doing gynecological surgery, recovering from being on call twenty-four hours straight, and trying to maintain a life outside the office. During pregnancy and early labor you'll probably feel very strongly that you want your doctor and no one else to deliver your baby. However, as labor intensifies—trust me—you won't care as much. What's really important is that you have an alert, prepared doctor who—especially at night—is well rested and able to focus on caring for you. Like me and thousands of other mothers before me, at the end of the day, you'll be absolutely fine with having a qualified person delivering your baby into your arms.

Patients sometimes stare at me blankly when I tell them that I might not be able to come in during the night, that I can't be yanked out of bed and be expected to make complex medical decisions. All of us have stories about the things we've done when exhausted, from the silly to downright frightening. When a physician is so tired after working long hours that basic routines—especially those affecting personal safety—are forgotten, it's time to hang up the stethoscope and get some sleep.

—JIM N., OB

- **Charge nurse.** This nurse is responsible for making sure things run smoothly throughout her eight- to twelve-hour shift. Charge nurses typically don't care directly for patients but make themselves available to assist nurses, patients, and families as needed. If for some reason you feel that your current labor and delivery nurse isn't a great match, or you want to make a switch for any other reason, the charge nurse is the person to speak with. She's also a good resource for other special requests/needs.
- **Pediatrician.** This is a medical doctor who specializes in taking care of infants and children. You should research and select a pediatrician during your pregnancy, *not* after the baby is born. When you arrive at the hospital in labor, the nurses will ask you who your baby's doctor is. The hospital will notify the pediatrician that the baby has been born, and he or she will be in to do a head-to-toe assessment within a few hours of delivery and once a day before you leave the hospital. The pediatrician is responsible for discharging the baby from the hospital and will tell you at that time when to bring your baby in for the first office visit (usually within the first week of birth). They'll be monitoring the baby's weight, skin color, etc., and will check to see how *you're* doing!

  If your pediatrician's office isn't close to the hospital where you'll be delivering, there's a possibility that he or she will not have privileges to practice there. In this situation, an in-house pediatrician will care for your baby throughout your stay in the same way your own pediatrician would. The in-house doc will also discharge the baby and will provide you with all the paperwork your own pediatrician needs—essentially a snapshot of the baby's first few days of life in the hospital, including the results of any testing, immunizations, and so on.

- **Lactation/breastfeeding consultant.** Because breastfeeding provides so many wonderful health benefits to your baby, it's important that you start as soon as possible. Babies are designed to be awake and alert for the first several hours after birth, so anytime in this window is perfect to introduce them to the breast and help them latch on for the first time. (After those first few hours, babies go into a deep sleep, which makes it harder to accomplish that first feeding.) Even after a cesarean birth, the hospital team will work diligently to get the baby to Mom in the recovery room so she can initiate breastfeeding. Labor and delivery and postpartum nurses are very capable of assisting you with breastfeeding. Be prepared, however, to hear all sorts of conflicting opinions on every aspect of breastfeeding, from everyone you know. Taking a good breastfeeding class prenatally will help you filter through all that advice.

  Unfortunately, getting Baby's mouth and Mom's nipple to work together isn't always as easy as you might think—especially when it's her first child. That's when it's time to contact a lactation consultant, whose job is to help you overcome the common challenges associated with breastfeeding.

  A lactation consultant will have one or more of the following credentials: CLE (certified lactation educator), CLC (certified lactation consultant), or IBCLC (International Board Certified Lactation Consultant), which means she has had literally thousands of hours of specialized education and training in the area of babies and breasts and everything in between. In addition, she may or may not be an RN.

  Whatever her credentials, one thing is for sure: She absolutely lives to see babies successfully breastfeed and strongly believes that breast milk is the best form of nutrition to get babies off to a healthy start in life. McMoyler Method agrees.

Most lactation consultants today also share our viewpoint that it's the milk that's important and not necessarily the route. If a mom finds that breastfeeding is too arduous, too painful, or too difficult for whatever reason, there's a great alternative: a breast pump. It's not necessarily more convenient, but it's another way to provide your baby with breast milk.

In many hospitals, on-staff lactation consultants make the rounds in the postpartum units, providing their expert assistance. However, since breastfeeding challenges really start cropping up when the baby is four to five days old (*after* you're out of the hospital), you may need to get some breastfeeding support at home. We recommend that you have the name and phone number of a good lactation consultant or lactation center already identified and included in your important-phone-numbers list on the refrigerator at home. Do it now, before labor starts. You'll be glad you did.

- **Anesthesiologist.** These are among the most highly trained physicians in the hospital. Their specialty is twofold: providing pain relief and, to put it bluntly, making sure their patients keep breathing. They are wildly popular in Labor and Delivery, and they split their time between placing labor epidurals, administering anesthesia during cesareans, and sometimes attending vaginal deliveries to make an initial assessment of the newborn. If you have an uncomplicated, intervention-free labor and delivery, you may not see an anesthesiologist at all. If you choose to have an epidural or spinal, he or she will assess your level of pain, make an in-depth review of your medical chart, take a medical history (including your overall health, previous surgeries, and allergies), and briefly explain the procedure. Once the medication starts to flow and you're comfortable, the anesthesiologist will be in and out of the room to check your progress and to adjust the dosage, as necessary. (If you need a cesarean, the anesthesiologist will handle any and all anesthesia-related issues. Besides managing the anesthesia for Mom, anesthesiologists are typically very good at keeping both expectant parents apprised of exactly what's going on and what to expect throughout the surgery.)

Note: Anesthesiologists are not the only medical professionals who administer anesthetics. Nurse anesthetists, for example, administer as much as 60 percent of anesthetics in the United States. The difference between a nurse anesthetist and an anesthesiologist is that the latter has a medical degree and has been through an anesthesia residency. A nurse anesthetist has a bachelor's degree in nursing, extensive critical-care experience, and a three-year master's degree in nursing anesthesia.

Nonepidural medication, such as narcotics, typically is administered by nurses, and local anesthesia (to the perineum) will be given by the OB or midwife.

- **OB technician.** This person is trained to scrub (assist and pass instruments) during a cesarean and may help out with other jobs in the labor and delivery unit.
- **Lab technician.** May be in to collect blood samples—a standard procedure in most hospitals. Sometimes this is done long before labor; other times the hospital may need additional blood drawn as labor progresses or when the decision to have a cesarean is made.
- **Unit secretary.** Although it's unlikely that this person will actually come into your labor room, she may very well be

the first person you meet when you arrive in Labor and Delivery. Unit secretaries work at the nurses' station and are kind of like the behind-the-scenes directors of the entire labor and delivery environment. They're very resourceful and know how to quickly locate anything or anyone you need.

- **Housekeeper.** This person will be in and out of your room, emptying the garbage and the linen hampers and restocking supplies. There will also be a certain amount of tidying and cleaning inside your room while you're still in it. Once you've delivered, the housekeepers will swarm into the room to clean and disinfect it from top to bottom.
- **Medical students.** Typically found in teaching or university hospitals, medical students are carefully monitored as they learn and practice different procedures. It's up to you whether they provide care to you. If you would rather they didn't, say so. No one will think any worse of you. They're usually very motivated to do a good job and are always closely supervised.
- **Family members or friends.** Before labor starts, it may seem like a great idea to invite all sorts of people you know and love to share in this momentous occasion. Try to resist the urge. For starters, when you first had this thought, you weren't in any pain and you weren't having one contraction after the other for hours on end. Think about the last time you had a bad case of the flu. Did you want a whole room full of people coming in and out to cheer you up? Probably not. The one you let near you to change the basin at the bedside, bring a fresh glass of water, and smooth the bedsheets was your husband, and no one else.

If you've already made the mistake of inviting your entire Rolodex and you have a change of heart at the hospital, your nurse will be happy to play the heavy. Just have your husband tell her that you need the room cleared and she'll take care of it. What if people show up in your labor room, unannounced and uninvited? Same strategy—the nurse will escort them out. The same goes for relatives. If you really want them to be there, that's okay, but you have every right to change your mind at any time. (Don't be too tough on them, though. Most visitors are just trying to be supportive—they aren't thinking about the fact that you've been up all night, pushed for two hours, and that all you really want is to get some sleep.)

A Note on Doulas

Although some couples have a doula with them throughout labor and delivery, it's important to remember that doulas are *not* medical professionals and, from the hospital's perspective, may not be completely welcome. Although I have a lot of respect for most doulas and what they do, I can see the hospital's point.

The problem is that some doulas have an agenda and see their role as protecting Mom and Baby from what they believe are unnecessary interventions. Sometimes they take that agenda a couple steps too far and start playing doctor, inserting their nonmedical opinion into a science-based hospital arena. As you can imagine, this can create tension and confusion, and is, frankly, completely inappropriate. In San Francisco, at least one major OB/GYN practice banned doulas from its delivery rooms after several of them persuaded patients to delay necessary procedures and interfered with the medical team's ability to do its job.

> *I really don't have any problem with doulas, just as long as they know their place—and that place is not between me and my patient. I've been delivering babies for more than twenty years and I think it's safe to say that I know a lot more about how to handle a delivery than a doula does.*
>
> —ROBERT Y., OB/GYN

One other potential problem: Having a doula almost guarantees that you'll be seeing a lot less of your labor and delivery nurse than you otherwise would. When you think about it, that makes perfect sense. If the doula is there doing part of the nurse's job, the nurse will spend more time with patients who need her more. In addition, there's a good chance that even when the nurses *are* there, the quality of care you get will be somewhat disjointed. Nurses base a lot of their decisions about what you need on talking with you and closely evaluating how you're coping with labor. If a doula is there, the nurse may not be able to establish a close enough connection with you to accurately assess the situation.

If you're committed to hiring a doula to go to the hospital with you, we strongly advise that you do the following:

- Get a recommendation from your OB or midwife. She'll have a short list of doulas she's worked with who are very good at what they do.
- Confirm with the prospective doula that she shares your reality-based view of the labor and birth process (meaning that flexibility is key).
- Have her come with you to at least one prenatal visit. It's essential that the doula and your OB/midwife have a chance to meet. You want to be proactive in avoiding delivery-room conflicts.

- Have her meet your husband at least once. He can then be the one to introduce her to the labor and delivery nurses, which will help create a tension-free environment.
- Make sure she understands that her role is to provide support for you *and* your husband, and she can stay with you if your husband needs to take a break outside the delivery room. Unfortunately, sometimes having a doula there can edge Dad out of center stage, which is where he really should be, providing the kind of unconditional love and support you need. So be very clear in communicating your needs to her—she's there to provide emotional support to both of you.

If the unexpected occurs during labor, and you find that you don't need or want the doula to continue with you, thank her and send her a check after you get home.

Sounds Kind of Crowded in There . . .

I know the list of medical professionals sounds quite long. Fortunately, you'll be seeing only a few of them at a time, depending on the situation.

- **Vaginal birth, no/low intervention** (which could include external monitoring and possibly an IV). During labor, you'll typically see one labor and delivery nurse per shift. Your OB/midwife will be in and out throughout labor and will stay for the delivery. After the baby is born, a nurse from the newborn nursery may come in to assess the baby. Otherwise, the labor and delivery nurse will care for both Baby and Mom from labor through recovery.

- **Vaginal birth with epidural.** Same as above, plus an anesthesiologist who, depending on the hospital, may make the initial assessment of the newborn.
- **Cesarean birth.** Six or seven people, not including you and your husband. The OB/primary surgeon, a second OB as assisting surgeon, a scrub nurse, a circulating nurse, an anesthesia provider (either an anesthesiologist or a nurse anesthetist), a pediatrician, and sometimes an intensive care nursery nurse.
- **Multiples.** If you're having two or more babies, the above numbers can easily be doubled. You'll have one to three physicians and one to two nurses, and each baby will have one to two physicians and at least one nurse.

SEEING DOUBLE

Twins (or more) are considered a high-risk pregnancy. For the most part, you can follow the guidelines we've talked about elsewhere in this chapter. There are, however, a few small but important differences.

- When you call to report that your water has broken, you'll be told to come in right away, regardless of whether you've started having contractions. (With a singleton your OB or midwife might have you stay at home for a while longer.)
- When you get to the hospital, plan on being continuously monitored to ensure that you and the babies are all tolerating labor. In most cases you'll still be able to be up and out of bed.
- You'll have an IV. If this occurs early in labor, you may want to inquire about having it "capped" off with a saline or heparin lock. This will allow you to stay mobile, while still providing IV access in case you need it later (most likely for an epidural).
- You may be pushing in more than one place. In many hospitals you'll begin in the labor room and at some point be moved down the hall to the OR, where you'll continue. The logic is that once Baby A is born vagi-

nally, if Baby B needs to be born by cesarean, you're already where you need to be and everything is set up and ready to go. Fortunately, obstetricians are much more aggressive these days with helping get Baby B into position for a vaginal birth. This has decreased the number of second-baby cesareans significantly.

- Be prepared for a crowd at the time of delivery! There will be a large team of medical professionals gathered to make sure all needs are met.

Talking the Talk

Okay, now that you know who's going to be there and what they're doing, let's listen in on what they're saying. Here are some of the terms and phrases you're likely to hear during labor, delivery, and right afterward.

Abnormal presentation. Ideally, your baby's first view of the world will be your OBs shoes (this is assuming you'll be delivering on your back). An abnormal presentation could be coming out leading with the chin, or looking at the ceiling (which could also be called a persistent posterior position; OP, for *occiput posterior;* or "sunny side up").

Abruptio placentae. When the placenta prematurely detaches from the wall of the uterus. This is a serious problem because the oxygen source to the baby can be acutely diminished. Mom may experience pain, her abdomen may feel rigid to the touch, and there may be bleeding. This condition results in an immediate cesarean delivery.

Amniotic fluid. This is the fluid inside the *amniotic sac,* which cushions and protects the fetus.

Analgesia. Pain-relieving medication.

Apgar score. A rating or score given to newborns at one, five, and sometimes again at ten minutes of age. The score is based on five categories: heart rate, respiratory rate, flexion, muscle tone, and color. The baby is given a score of 0 to 2 for each category. By the five-minute mark, most will have a score of 8–9. In theory, all brand-new babies should have a point deducted for color, as it takes up to a week for their blood to start circulating through the body efficiently. Babies whose Apgar score is below 7 at five minutes will go to the nursery for further evaluation.

Assisted delivery. An attempt to facilitate delivery—the two most common approaches are forceps and vacuum extractors. See the chart on page 144 for more.

Breech presentation. The baby is trying to come out butt or feet first, instead of head first. This almost always results in a scheduled cesarean delivery.

Cardinal movements. This is the corkscrewing motion the baby does as it descends toward the exit sign (it's similar to the twisting and turning you have to do to get your rings off your fingers). Many babies who are in the "undesirable" posterior position early in labor will eventually turn into the desired (anterior) position, thanks to the effects of cardinal movements.

Cephalopelvic disproportion. The baby's head is too large to fit through the mother's pelvis. Requires a cesarean.

Cervix. The necklike lower part of the uterus that dilates and thins in response to uterine contractions and allows the baby to pass.

Cord compression. This is when the cord is wrapped around the baby's neck, looped around the body, or wedged between the baby's head and the mother's pelvis. When the cord is compressed, blood circulation is decreased and the baby's heart rate can drop. Intermittent monitoring throughout labor and continuous monitoring while pushing has revolutionized our ability to identify these situations. Compression can sometimes be relieved by having Mom change positions. If that doesn't resolve the problem, a cesarean may be required.

Crowning. The appearance of the infant's head at the vaginal opening and "+4 station." You are now only moments away from meeting your baby.

Dilation. The gradual opening of the neck of the cervix to permit passage of the baby into the vagina. Dilation is measured in centimeters. One centimeter is about the size of a Cheerio; 5 centimeters is the size of a vanilla wafer; 10 centimeters is the size of a good-quality bagel.

Effacement. The gradual thinning, shortening, and drawing up of the cervix. Effacement is measured in percentages from 0 (no thinning) to 100 (completely thinned out).

Engaged. This means that the baby is at the bottom of the pelvis, in a spot that's also called "zero station." At this point, most women are actively pushing the baby into the birth canal.

Episiotomy. A surgical incision made into the perineum (the area between the vagina and anus) that enlarges the vaginal opening for delivery of the baby. The incision is repaired with stitches after the baby and placenta have been delivered. See page 151 for more.

Fetal distress/fetal intolerance of labor. This is when information from fetal monitoring suggests that the baby is no longer tolerating the labor or pushing. In this situation, decisions may need to be made very quickly, with little time for discussion.

Fetal heart rate monitor. A device (internal or external) that tracks and records the baby's heart rate throughout labor and delivery.

Induction. The use of medication (prostaglandins and/or Pitocin) to get labor started. (Acupuncture is also recognized as sometimes being successful in helping labor begin.)

Intrauterine. Inside the uterus.

Involution. The process of the uterus returning to its normal size after delivery.

Lightening. The process of the baby "dropping" as it descends toward the pelvic cavity.

Local anesthesia. Numbing the perineum with anesthetic medication. Unlike a spinal or epidural, which numbs large sections of the body, locals numb very small areas, in the same way a dentist numbs a small area of your mouth before drilling.

Lochia. The discharge from the uterus that occurs after both vaginal and cesarean births. Days one through three will be a heavy flow, days three through five moderate, becoming gradually lighter over the next two to four weeks.

Pelvic exam. These vaginal exams provide essential information to your medical team about your progress in labor. See "The Ins and Outs of Vaginal Exams" on page 140 for more.

Perineal tear. If the tissue between the vagina and anus can't stretch enough to allow the baby to be delivered, it may tear and need to be stitched. See page 151 for more.

Pitocin. The synthetic version of a natural hormone called *oxytocin.* Pitocin stimulates contractions and can be given to induce or augment labor. You may also get it after the delivery to help the uterine muscle to contract, which constricts the blood vessels, thereby preventing unnecessary bleeding.

Placenta. The flat, circular organ in the pregnant uterus that serves as the exchange station for nutrients and oxygen that move from mother to baby. The placenta is delivered after the baby and is often referred to as the afterbirth. In a vaginal delivery it takes an average of five to fifteen minutes for the placenta to separate from the wall of the uterus and to then be pushed out. In a cesarean birth, the placenta is manually removed from the uterus after the baby has been delivered.

Placenta previa. When the placenta is attached to the uterus too low or is completely covering the opening of the cervix. It can cause bleeding during the pregnancy, premature birth (infrequently), and is often an indication for a scheduled cesarean.

Postpartum. The time period immediately after the birth. Most people consider the postpartum period to last about six weeks, since that's about when a new mom will go back to see her OB/midwife for a postpartum checkup. McMoyler Method emphasizes that the six-week definition can be very misleading. The reality is that it takes many months, if not a year, for the body to completely heal and for the couple to fully adapt, adjust, and settle into parenthood.

Prolapsed cord. This is when the umbilical cord slides out of the cervix before the baby does. When the uterus contracts to push the baby down, pressure on the cord can diminish blood flow to the baby. (There is sometimes a connection between prolapsed cord and the amniotic sac rupturing. If the baby's head is still high, there's a slim chance that the rush of fluid could carry the cord down in front of the head.) May require an emergency cesarean.

Pudendal block. See "local anesthesia" above.

Station. This is an indication of how far the baby has traveled through the pelvis, measured in centimeters. A negative number ("–2 station") means that the head hasn't entered the pelvis. Zero station (also called "engaged") means that the baby's head is inside the pelvis. A positive number ("+1 station") means that the head is starting to come down into the pelvis. Crowning occurs at +4 station.

Transverse lie. When the baby is in the womb in a horizontal position.

Umbilical cord. This is the internal lifeline for the unborn baby. It connects the baby to the placenta and delivers oxygenated blood and nutrition from the mother to the baby. After delivery, the cord is cut by the OB, midwife, or partner. The stump dries up and on average falls off in about ten days, although it could take as long as two to three weeks. Since there are no nerve endings in the cord, the cutting, drying, and healing don't cause the baby any pain or discomfort.

We Now Interrupt This Birth . . .

We've all heard the stories about how pregnant women (usually in other cultures) would be working in a field, go into labor, have

DadBox

The Ins and Outs of Vaginal Exams (aka Pelvic Exams)

Guys, you're going to have to trust me on this one: There isn't a woman on earth who looks forward to pelvic exams—in fact, they're what most women dread most about their annual physical (mammograms are also high on the list). Sometime during the last trimester, starting at around thirty-six weeks, she will probably have one at every prenatal visit. (The purpose is to see whether her body has started to prepare for labor with some effacement or initial dilation.) Once she's in labor, it's going to seem like she's having a pelvic every hour (although in reality it's a lot less frequent). Plus, when the baby is still "riding high" and hasn't started to move its way down the birth canal, it can feel as if the nurse or doctor is trying to examine her tonsils! The reality is that this is the only way to accurately determine the progress of labor.

So why am I telling you this? Simple: because your wife and the nursing staff can really use your help. When she's wound up tight as a clock (and most laboring women are), teeth clenched, shoulders tense, knees locked, it's really hard to perform the exam and gather the necessary information.

Here's how you can make those inevitable exams more doable. If you aren't already there, move to the head of the bed. Then get in her face and do what you would do if she were between contractions: remind her to release and let go, give her specific cues like "drop your shoulders," "take a long, deep breath," "unclench your teeth," and "uncurl your toes." Keep in mind, you do not need to spend any time at the south end of the bed unless you want to. With you there to help, these pelvic exams can move from difficult to manageable.

their baby, and be back on the job in a couple of hours. To the extent that was ever true, I can't imagine that anyone would want to return to those times. Today there's hardly an aspect of pregnancy, labor, or delivery where Western medicine hasn't gotten involved. In the chart that follows, I'll tell you about the most common medical interventions, what's involved, how prevalent they are, and how they're used to manage labor. Chances are, you'll encounter at least a few of these interventions, so arming yourself with as much information about them as possible will help you better evaluate your options and make more informed decisions.

There are three important interventions that we need to spend a little more time on:

- Induction
- Epidural
- Cesarean

If you don't know what's going on around you, it's easy to feel apprehensive or frightened, or to worry that something is being pushed on you, so let's go through them step by step. Having a good understanding of these procedures will enable you and your partner to have more in-depth discussions with your health care team about your options.

Induction

The average pregnancy lasts forty weeks. Once you pass that estimated due date, your physician or midwife will probably raise the issue of inducing labor. Why? Because starting at about forty weeks, a number of things start to happen:

Common Interventions

Name	What it is and when it's used
External fetal monitoring	• This routine procedure involves placing two monitors on your records the baby's heart rate, while the contraction monitor tracks your contractions (but not the strength). • You'll be monitored an average of once every hour during labor, (although some OBs may prefer continuous monitoring). • Some form of external monitoring has been the norm since the information was gathered by hand. Today it's done by machine superior and more efficient.
Intravenous fluids	• The benefits of an IV include hydration throughout labor as well as medication or antibiotics. • If you have a labor narcotic or an epidural you will need to have • If the IV is not needed continuously, ask about having it capped off This will eliminate the need (for the time being) for the tubing, bag, • When labor goes on for a long time, the fluids you're getting by completely replenish what you're using. The IV enables you to get for you, sometimes it's for the baby. • IV hydration often helps restore a stalled labor pattern. Like a sometimes perk up with some extra fluid. And that may eliminate interventions.
Amniotomy (artificial rupture of membranes, or AROM)	• Also called "snagging the bag" • If the amniotic sac has not ruptured on its own, your physician (using an amniohook to do the manual rupturing) to help labor color of the amniotic fluid. • The fluid should be clear to straw colored but on occasion may baby's first stool. • If the fluid is meconium-stained, you may require internal monitoring, specialists will be brought in for the delivery. They will carefully and provide additional suctioning to clear out any remaining
Restrictions on food and drink	Some hospitals require that women stop eating solids and switch are admitted and/or are in active labor. The idea is to keep the that general anesthesia would be used.
Systemic analgesia	Fast-acting, short-lasting narcotics, discussed in greater detail in
Regional anesthesia (aka epidural)	Discussed in greater detail in Chapter 2, as well as below
Local anesthesia	Given by injection into the perineal area (between the rectum and repair a tear

	Risks	How common?
abdomen. The fetal monitor the frequency and duration of and continuously while pushing 1960s. Before then, the same because the technology is far	None	Almost universal
providing a way to administer an IV in place first. with a saline or heparin lock. and pole. mouth are often not enough to a bigger "drink." Sometimes it's wilted flower, a tired uterus can the need for more aggressive	Might restrict mobility but doesn't have to. Just about the only place she may not be able to be is in the shower, and some nurses will help you accomplish even that.	80–90%
may suggest an amniotomy progress and/or to assess the contain meconium, which is the and additional health care examine the baby's airways meconium.	• Infection • Prolapsed cord	About 50% of women have AROM. That percentage goes up if the baby is overdue.
over to clear liquids when they stomach empty in the rare case	There is some controversy about whether to completely restrict or simply minimize intake of solids. Ask your OB or midwife how this is handled at your hospital.	This is considered standard
Chapter 2, Pain Realities		20–40%
		70–80% Lower in rural areas, higher in urban ones
the vagina) for episiotomy or to		+/-15%

(continues)

Common Interventions *(continued)*

Name	What it is and when it's used
Internal fetal monitoring	• Internal monitoring is used to obtain more accurate heart rate baby is tolerating labor and pushing. • A small electrode is inserted through the birth canal and attached • The bag of waters must have already ruptured for this monitor to
Oxygen	• Generally delivered via nasal prongs or a face mask • Most often used to provide the baby with increased oxygen
Foley catheter	• Tube inserted through the urethra, up into the bladder • Used to keep the bladder empty during a cesarean or with an
Intrauterine pressure catheter (IUPC)	• Like a tire pressure gauge, this catheter is used to measure the • It's inserted vaginally and guided through the opening of the uterine wall and the baby's head. • It's sometimes used to introduce saline into the uterus to dilute
Vacuum extractor	• A suction cup is placed on the baby's head to help guide it down physician will pull on the vacuum handle while the uterus contracts an average of only four contractions. • You must have already pushed the baby to a +2 station for • The baby's heart rate is continuously monitored to ensure that he's • After birth, there may be a bruise on the top of the baby's head, cup was attached will be puffy. Both will fade within a few days.
Forceps delivery	• Tongs-like instruments used while you're pushing to assist the baby birth canal. Like vacuum extractors, forceps are used for an and you will have to have pushed the baby to +2 station before • "Salad spoons" are inserted through the vagina around the baby's along the baby's jawline and clasp into place. While the uterus carefully guides the baby to crowning • The baby's heart rate is continuously monitored to ensure that he
Episiotomy	See the sidebar on page 151 for more.
Augmentation	• You're already in labor and uterine contractions have slowed. IV back the strength and frequency of contractions. • In some cases, the stalled labor may be caused by an epidural.

	Risks	How common?
information, confirming that the to the baby's scalp. be used.	• May require episiotomy • Slightly increased incidence of infection Usually requires an episiotomy	+/-10%
		Many patients will get oxygen at some point in the process, either toward the end of labor, during pushing, and always during a cesarean.
epidural.	Possible irritation to urethra. Infection is rare.	Standard with epidural and cesarean
actual strength of contractions. cervix. It then rests between the meconium-stained fluid		+/-25%
through the birth canal. The and Mom pushes. It's used for vacuum to be used. tolerating the procedure and the areas where the suction	• Cephalohemotoma (bruising) • Increased chance of developing jaundice • Possible laceration or blistering • May require episiotomy	+/-15–20 %
through the lower part of the average of four contractions, they can be used. head, one at a time. They fit contracts and you push, the OB is tolerating the procedure.		+/-5%
	Potential for increased tearing, infection, incontinence, discomfort during sexual intercourse.	25–30%
Pitocin is administered to bring	Hyperstimulation. Requires continuous monitoring to evaluate fetal heart rate and contractions.	More common with first labors

- Amniotic fluid levels go down.
- The placenta starts aging and doesn't do its job as well as it used to.
- The baby keeps on getting bigger, which makes delivery more challenging. (From thirty-six weeks on, pretty much all the baby does is put on weight. Beware of the Häagen-Dazs baby!)

If you haven't gone into labor on your own by forty weeks, your health care provider will begin discussing induction with you. At forty-one weeks, he or she will schedule a date for you to be admitted to the hospital to induce labor. (If you've been diagnosed with gestational diabetes or elevated blood pressure, your doctor may suggest inducing before then.)

Here's how a typical induction will unfold:

You'll arrive at the hospital in the late afternoon or early evening *before* the actual date of induction. There usually aren't any dietary restrictions to observe prior to an induction (although you should check with your doctor just to make sure), so you and your partner can go out for a nice meal beforehand.

Once you check in, the rest of the evening will be devoted to coaxing the cervix to soften, shorten, or efface. In some instances, it may begin to dilate, although that isn't the expectation.

This process, which I call "priming the pump," is accomplished with the help of a synthetic form of *prostaglandin* (a normally occurring hormone that causes labor to begin). These synthetic prostaglandins come in tablet or gel form, either one of which will be inserted vaginally and tucked up by the cervix. The results can range from mildly irritating to quite uncomfortable. Some women will respond with crampiness; others will actually begin having

DadBox

If your wife is being induced, do not drop her off at the hospital and head back home. Oh, no. You should plan on spending the night there. There's no way to know exactly how she's going to respond to this evening of pump priming. It might be a relaxing evening in front of the tube, or she might start having contractions, which could catch her completely off-guard. That's rare, but if it happens, she'll need you to be there. Even if labor doesn't start, she'll really appreciate the emotional support. A tip: If you and/or your wife want to shower in the morning, tell your night nurse so she can make sure you're up early enough to finish before the actual induction begins.

contractions. You'll be continuously monitored and in bed for several hours, and depending on your progress, you might need to have repeated doses throughout the night.

The next morning, your nurse will arrive early (usually between 6 and 7 a.m.) to start an IV, which will remain in place until your baby is born. The nurse will then begin administering Pitocin to cause uterine contractions. The Pitocin will be delivered in very small, incremental doses via a continuous pump. Your nurse will increase the dose every twenty to thirty minutes, until you're having contractions every two minutes that last sixty seconds. Achieving this goal could take anywhere from a few hours to two days. (A two-day induction is not standard, but it could happen.)

During the induction, continuous monitoring is the standard of care in most hospitals, as they need to be sure that the baby is tolerating the induction process and receiving an adequate break in between contractions, and to confirm that there are in fact enough contractions to cause you to go into labor. In other hospitals, patients may be taken off the monitors in early labor.

The vast majority of women who are induced will at some point choose an epidural. The main reason is that most inductions are done for large or overdue babies. It typically takes more contractions and a longer labor to give birth to a large baby, and as the length of labor increases, so does the need for an epidural.

The main difference between contractions caused by oxytocin during spontaneous labor and those caused by Pitocin during induced labor is the way they feel. If you ask a woman who has had synthetically induced contractions, she'll tell you that they shoot up to the peak very quickly (which leaves little or no time to get ready), stay there for what feels like a looong time, and then drop back just as suddenly (which doesn't leave much time for recovery). In a labor that unfolds on its own, contractions build steadily, peak, then slowly subside. This gives Mom a chance to prepare on the way up, endure the twenty- to forty-second peak, and then recover on the way down. It's important to note, though, that this situation is changing. When Pitocin is administered slowly and thoughtfully, induced labor can progress very much like spontaneous labor, and studies of intrauterine pressure catheters show no difference between the two types of contractions.

The following interventions could accompany an induction in conjunction with an epidural. See pages 142–145 for more.

- Intrauterine pressure catheter to measure the strength of contractions
- Fetal scalp electrode to more closely monitor the baby's heart rate
- A Foley catheter to empty your bladder

- An automatic blood pressure cuff to continuously monitor your blood pressure
- Oxygen via face mask or nasal prongs

Epidurals

Epidural anesthesia is the most common form of regional anesthesia used during labor. Since the entire procedure is done behind you, you won't be able to see anything that's happening. It's definitely worthwhile to know what's going on, so here's a description of the way a typical epidural is done and how you'll be affected before, during, and after the procedure.

1. The anesthesiologist and nurse will help you get into a position that helps locate the right spot on your lower back to place the epidural catheter (between two of your lower lumbar vertebrae). You may be lying down, curled into a fetal position, or sitting up and leaning over the bedside table. Many women are concerned that they won't be able to hold still during a contraction. Your nurse will be right there every minute to help you. Your partner may be there for additional support. The anesthesiologist will talk you through what you need to do and will stop as often as possible to allow you to move through the contraction. In my experience, women who choose epidurals are very motivated to hold still—relief is on the way.
2. The anesthesiologist will inject a local anesthetic to numb the spot. Once you're numb, a needle will be inserted in between the vertebrae into the epidural space, which is the space closest to the outside of the body, meaning that they

do not have to go as deep. A very thin, flexible plastic catheter will be passed through this needle. Then the needle will be removed and the catheter will stay behind, taped to your back so it won't come out.

3. The anesthesiologist delivers a test dose to ensure that he has located just the right place to administer the epidural medication. He will then deliver an anesthetic mixed with a narcotic through the catheter. Within fifteen minutes, you'll be partially numb from the waist down. (A well-functioning epidural replaces pain with a sense of pressure.)
4. Typically, a *continuous infusion pump* is placed next to the labor bed. This pump will deliver a consistent amount of medication throughout. In response to your individual needs, the anesthesiologist will adjust the dosage of medication to keep you numb throughout labor and into the pushing stage.
5. Once your epidural is in place, you won't be able to eat or drink anything besides small sips of water and ice chips.

Although people talk about epidurals as if they're a standalone procedure, they usually lead to a cascade of other interventions, including some of the ones listed below. There's no guarantee that you'll need all of them, but we recommend that you familiarize yourself with what they are and how they're used, and discuss any questions with your OB or midwife.

- Intravenous fluids
- Automatic blood pressure cuff to monitor your blood pressure
- A Foley catheter to drain your bladder
- Pitocin to keep labor progressing

TO CUT OR NOT TO CUT . . .

In the last century, episiotomies were routine, and almost every expectant mom had one. Today, it's in your doctor's (and your) best interest *not* to have one. Most experts agree that a minimal amount of perineal tearing is preferable to an episiotomy. Perineal tissue that separates naturally from the pressure of the baby's head will heal more efficiently than an incision will. As for your doctor, if he's able to deliver your baby over an intact perineum, he'll be finished with his job, congratulating you, and out the door far sooner than if he had to stay around and suture up an incision.

The episiotomy decision is made on a case-by-case basis—it's only when the baby is beginning to crown that the doctor can determine whether the perineum will stretch enough to allow the head out without creating a severe tear. Years ago, doctors cut a one-size-fits-all episiotomy. Today physicians make the smallest incision possible to allow the baby's head to come out. If your doctor suspects that there will be significant tearing, he'll probably opt for the episiotomy as a way to control and protect the perineum. (And just so you know, if you have an epidural, your doctor will test the numbness in the perineum before cutting. If you don't have an epidural, you'll get an injection of a local anesthetic to numb the whole area.)

Because neither a tear nor an episiotomy is a particularly desirable option, McMoyler Method recommends two steps that have helped many women avoid both.

1. Apply warm compresses to the perineum during pushing. This will usually be done by the nurse and can be started when the baby's head first comes into view (which is quite a bit ahead of crowning). The warm compress (a washcloth dipped in warm water and wrung out) can be applied to the perineum during the contraction, while Mom is pushing, and she can be encouraged with a visual image of "pushing toward the warm."
2. The nurse or doctor can do perineal massage during the pushing stage and while the head is crowning. They'll use either warm oil that's stocked in the labor and delivery unit or simply use vaginal secretions.

The warmth and moisture from the compresses and the massage will increase blood flow to the perineum, which increases elasticity and allows the tissue to stretch a bit more. Even the tiniest amount of extra stretch can help keep the perineum intact.

While avoiding an episiotomy is a great goal, keep in mind that this is one of those delivery-related decisions that have to be made in the moment. I strongly suggest that you turn the decision-making over to the person at the foot of the bed. Your OB/midwife is in the driver's seat now, assessing and calculating, using his knowledge and experience to make the best decision on your behalf. If the OB anticipates a nasty tear, he'll probably cut an episiotomy. Or he may let the baby's emerging head stay at +4 crowning for a few extra moments to further help the tissues stretch. (This brief pause is referred to as "the ring of fire"—and in the not-too-distant future, you'll know exactly why.) Similarly, if your OB tells you *not* to push with the next contraction, he's giving the tissues even more time to stretch by letting the contraction do the work of moving the baby slowly over the perineum.

An important note on perineal massage: Many childbirth classes and books still recommend that couples do perineal massage toward the end of the pregnancy. Although there's certainly no harm in doing this, understand that it will have absolutely zero effect on whether you have an episiotomy. Perineal massage is effective in preventing an episiotomy *only* when the perineal tissues are undergoing the kind of stretch experienced during crowning.

- Fetal scalp electrode to more closely monitor the baby's heart rate
- Intrauterine pressure catheter to accurately assess the strength of your contractions

Despite what you may have heard, it's never too late—physiologically—to have an epidural. You can, however, run out of time. What I mean is that if you decide very late in labor that you want an epidural, there may not be enough time to get the procedure done. By the time the anesthesiologist has been notified, you sign your consent forms, get adequate IV fluids, are positioned and prepped, and the medication has been injected into the epidural space, at least thirty minutes will have passed. At that point, you'll probably be ready to push the baby out—something most women describe as more doable than coping with labor contractions.

> **DadBox**
>
> You spent an impressive amount of time preparing for the birth of your baby, learning and understanding the various ways you can help your wife cope with her pain and bring your baby into the world. And then she has an epidural. It's tempting to think that if there's no pain to help her through, you've just been put out of a job. Not at all. You've still got a big role to play. Please review the section on pages 90–91 that discusses exactly what you can and should be doing from the time the epidural procedure starts.

Potential Risks Associated with Epidurals

In the right situation, an epidural can be the perfect choice. It provides complete relaxation and allows the cervix to open and the baby to descend. At the same time, though, there are some risks you should be aware of.

- **Blood pressure.** A drop in blood pressure is the most common side effect of epidural anesthesia. To minimize this risk, you'll receive 1 to 2 liters of IV fluids before the procedure even begins, which helps maintain your blood pressure. From the beginning of the epidural procedure until the baby is a few hours old, you'll have an automatic blood pressure cuff on your upper arm, which will fire off every five to fifteen minutes, squeezing down as it reads your blood pressure. It's a little annoying, but a fair trade-off for the pain. If your pressure does drop, the anesthesiologist will inject another medication to immediately raise it.

- **Shaking.** This is temporary and is best relieved with slow, deep breathing, which your husband can do with you. Another solution is to give you another medication through your IV.
- **Nausea.** Treated with an antinausea medication injected into your IV.
- **Effect on labor.** Old-style epidurals were notorious for slowing down progress—particularly when given early on—by causing contractions to spread out. In some cases, epidurals were thought to hinder pushing efforts, making delivery of the baby's head more difficult. However, today's lower-dose, patient-controlled epidurals are less likely to slow the frequency of labor contractions. Many health care professionals agree that epidurals may actually allow labor to proceed more effectively toward the pushing stage. Prior to the epidural, a combination of the pain you endured during contractions, plus increased tension and inability to relax *between* contractions, may have kept you from getting the rest you needed and stalled labor. Epidurals allow every muscle in your body to reach a limp-noodle state. That, in turn, allows you to rest—and maybe even sleep!—and build up the energy you'll need to push the baby out. Best of all, the relaxation of the pelvic floor during the crowning phase helps the baby's head descend and reduces the risk of tearing.
- **Ineffective pain relief.** Approximately 85 percent of women get total relief from epidurals. The other 15 percent experience only partial relief. This is referred to as having a "window on the uterus"—a section of the uterine muscle where the medication simply doesn't take. The choice is then to

gut it out with 3/4 relief or to start the procedure all over in an attempt to get complete relief.

- **Headache.** If the membrane that confines the spinal space is inadvertently punctured, a "higher-than-optimum" level of anesthetic may be absorbed, and a spinal headache may develop. This is usually relieved by analgesics, lying flat, and drinking fluids. In some cases, a "blood patch" (a small amount of the patient's own blood injected into the low back to seal the puncture that's causing the headache) will be performed before leaving the hospital. Less frequently, the patient may need to return to the hospital for this procedure. Either way, patients report almost instantaneous relief from what was an excruciating headache.
- **Infection.** Rare.
- **Nerve damage and paralysis.** *Extremely* rare.
- **Risk to the baby.** No direct risks, although the risks to the mom could inadvertently affect the baby.

Cesarean Birth

As we discussed in Chapter 5, on average, nearly 30 percent of babies in the United States are delivered by cesarean. Whether *you* have one will depend on a number of factors that fall into three general categories.

- Baby-related issues (explained in the chart of interventions on pages 135–139)
    - Cephalopelvic disproportion (head is too big to fit through the pelvis)
    - Fetal distress (baby is no longer tolerating labor or pushing, as seen via fetal heart rate monitoring)

    - Abnormal presentation (facing posterior is most common)
    - Breech presentation (feet or bottom first)
    - Transverse lie (lying horizontally)
- Placenta and umbilical cord issues (explained on pages 135–139)
    - Placenta previa
    - Abruptio placentae
    - Prolapsed cord
    - Cord compression
- Maternal indications, which may include:
    - Heart condition
    - Poorly controlled diabetes
    - Pregnancy-induced hypertension
    - High blood pressure
    - Active case of genital herpes
    - Multiple gestation (twins or more)
    - Prolonged rupture of membranes (more than twenty-four hours without any labor progress)
    - Failure to progress (meaning the cervix does not open beyond 3–4 centimeters)
    - The baby does not descend in station
    - Previous cesarean with vertical incision into the uterus
    - Maternal age (the older you are, the greater your chances of needing a cesarean)

Preparing for a Cesarean

If you are having a scheduled cesarean, you'll usually be admitted to the hospital the day of the procedure. The standard policy is no food for eight hours and no drink for six hours before the operation (although some hospitals may allow clear liquids up to three hours before). Your health care provider will fill you in on this and any other pre-operative instructions.

Leave all valuables at home, including rings, earrings, and necklaces. If you wear contacts, you'll need to remove them before the operation. You can, however, bring your glasses into the operating room (OR) with you.

Once you're admitted into your temporary room on the labor and delivery floor, you'll be pretty busy. Your baby's heart rate will be monitored, and your vital signs (temperature, blood pressure, etc.) will be taken. Your anesthesiologist will meet you, do a brief physical assessment, review your medical history, and discuss the anesthesia procedure. And your obstetrician will stop by, typically right before the scheduled time. In between, you'll have a big stack of paperwork, including consent forms, to review and sign.

Once that's all done, you'll get a small cup of sodium bi-citrate, which is used to neutralize the contents of your stomach. It's extremely salty and it's best to drink it down in one gulp. Your nurse will insert an IV into your arm and will shave your abdomen down to the top of the pubic hairline. Then you'll get a poofy paper bonnet to cover your head.

At this point you'll say a temporary goodbye to your partner. He'll get a paper outfit of his own (often called a bunny suit, for some reason that no one can remember) and will be shown where to wait outside the OR until you're fully prepped. If you already have an epidural in place, the anesthesiologist will use that to numb you. If you don't have an epidural, you could get a spinal. Spinals are frequently used in surgery and are an effective form of anesthesia. Your nurse will insert a Foley catheter into your bladder and will wash down your belly with a disinfectant and/or cover your entire abdomen with a drape that has a disinfectant built in.

You'll be lying on a very firm, narrow operating table, covered in flannel blankets from the thighs down, and literally strapped onto the table with a safety belt. Your arms usually will be loosely attached to arm boards to keep you from accidentally getting them into the sterile field. You'll have oxygen from either a face mask or nasal prongs, a *pulse oximeter* (which measures the amount of oxygen in your blood) on your index finger, and an automatic blood pressure cuff on your upper arm.

Finally, a drape will be placed across your body at chest level, and your partner will be brought in and seated on a stool next to your head. On the other side of the drape, a whole team of doctors and nurses will be working. There are two obstetricians (one is the primary surgeon, the other assists), one scrub nurse, one circulating nurse, and someone (either a nurse or an MD) from the nursery. If you're delivering twins, add at least two to four more doctors and/or nurses to the team.

EMERGENCY CESAREAN

Despite what you may have seen on television, true obstetrical emergencies are not common. In the rare situation when a mom is in trouble or a baby needs to be born, step out of the way of the health care team! They'll suddenly appear and will move the mom quickly into the OR. In these cases, general anesthesia is used to save on the time that would be needed to provide an adequate level of anesthesia from an epidural. Partners will not be in the OR (truth be told, the health care team can't deal with husbands right then; their focus is on the health of the mom and baby). He'll be pacing up and down the corridor burning a hole in the carpet, waiting to be told that his wife and baby are both fine.

Once the process has started, your baby will be lifted out of the womb within fifteen to twenty minutes (or, in the case of an emergency, as little as three minutes) and handed off in one fell swoop to the waiting arms of a pediatrician or a nursery nurse who will place the baby onto a warming table. (If you happen to smell smoke in the OR, don't worry. Chances are, it's the result of the surgeon cauterizing veins as he makes each incision through the layers of tissue down to the uterus.)

Hopefully, you and your partner will have discussed ahead of time what happens next. Does he accompany the baby to the nursery and meet you back in the recovery room, or does he stay with you while the medical team finishes up the cesarean? In this situation, your baby will go to the nursery and will join you and your partner in recovery a little later. (Hospitals generally won't allow you to keep the baby in the operating room during your entire surgery. The operating room has to be kept cool to control infection and that temperature is low for a newborn.)

Regardless of whether Dad and Baby stay with you, your medical team is still on the job. They'll be delivering the placenta

DadBox

While your wife is getting prepped for surgery, you'll get a "bunny suit," which is usually a one-piece paper jumpsuit that you wear right over your clothes. (Remember to empty your bladder before putting it on.) You'll also get a face mask, a poofy paper hat, and "booties," which are paper shoe covers. Cameras are okay (but be sure to ask before you tape the medical team; some may prefer not to be filmed). You'll have to wait outside the OR until your wife is fully prepped, then you can join her inside, where you'll be seated on a stool near her head.

After Baby is delivered, you can usually walk carefully over to the warming table, cut the remaining segment of cord, take some pictures, and bond for a few minutes. Once Baby is cleaned up and swaddled, he'll be taken to Mom for a few minutes, then it's off to the nursery. Ideally, the two of you will have decided long ago whether you'll stay with Mom or go to the nursery with Baby. If you haven't, do it *now.*

(manually, through the incision) and will spend thirty to forty-five minutes suturing all the layers back together. We'll discuss your postoperative recovery in more detail in Chapter 7.

A Very Important Note

If you weren't anticipating a cesarean, it's perfectly normal to have some feelings of disappointment. Please remember that you've just accomplished your goal—the birth of your baby! You are *not* a failure. We'll talk a lot more in Chapter 7 about avoiding (and overcoming) negative feelings like these.

Strategies for Success

As you know from the previous chapter, your medical team is on your side, and they'll do everything they can to help you have a safe and satisfying birth experience.

By reading this book, you've differentiated yourself and your husband from most of the other patients your nurses and doctors usually see. You're already familiar with the process of labor and delivery, you know the terminology, you understand that this journey is likely going to take some unexpected twists and turns before you reach the end, you're placing your trust in the professionals, and you're prepared to work with them to make decisions along the way. Now let's build on that foundation and discuss some specific strategies you can use to build a close working relationship with the medical team.

- **Be sure to take the hospital tour.** Taking the hospital tour will get you familiar with where to park, which entrance to use on weekdays versus weekends or night versus day, insurance updates, preregistration information, security information, the location of the waiting room for relatives, visiting hours, where the cafeteria is, and so on.

- **Pack your bags.** Have your hospital bags ready to go after thirty-six weeks. Chances are slim that you'll need them that early, but it's better to be on the safe side—just ask anyone who was caught off-guard by her water breaking or the sudden onset of labor. See our suggested packing lists on pages 69–70 for a list of what to bring. It's less than you might think.
- **Don't jump the gun and show up at the hospital after the first contraction.** Find out whom to call when you think it's time to go to the hospital. Is it your OB, or should you call Labor and Delivery, which will in turn call the doctor? Either way, you need to call *someone.* Do *not* just arrive on their doorstep. You want the red-carpet treatment: a nurse already assigned to you, your chart pulled, and a room ready and waiting. When you think that it's time to head out, call your OB, midwife, or the hospital before leaving, and do the walk/talk test (if she can walk and talk during a contraction, it's most likely too early to head for the hospital) we described in Chapter 4.
- **Remain calm if the equipment in the labor room starts beeping.** Your nurse will explain what it means. Often it's just an alarm indicating that the baby has moved into a position where the external monitor can't read the heartbeat. A simple repositioning of the monitor belts will usually take care of this. It could be that your wife's automatic blood pressure cuff needs adjusting, or maybe it's as basic as letting the nurse know that she needs to change the roll of paper in the bedside electronic monitor.

UNDERSTANDING HOSPITAL CULTURE

Like any other group of people, medical professionals come in a variety of shapes, sizes, and personalities. Depending on you as a couple, you may end up hitting it off with them right away, or you may need to help them understand your individual needs. During the delivery of our first son, Luke, our nurse was shy, but, boy, was she efficient, getting us what we needed quietly and quickly. With our second son, Corey, I remember that our nurse was animated and chatty. Ordinarily that doesn't bother me—I'm usually the most energetic person in the room—but I was feeling pretty bad, so I whispered to my husband to tell her that I needed quiet, now! Corey was born pretty soon after that, and I apologized to the nurse for being beyond crabby. She laughed and said, "Are you kidding? You did a great job!"

- **Remember, they're on your side.** Your nurses want to see progress in labor, they want to help you make decisions, and they want to end up with an intact, healthy family. Sounds like what you want, too, doesn't it?

  You can't imagine how many times I've seen couples come in with a stay-back-we-know-what-we're-doing-and-we-know-what-we-want attitude, prepared to defend themselves from the health care team. These couples act as if someone had warned them that *they* (whoever that is) would try to do things to the mom that she didn't want or need, that the medical staff would jump to interventions, that they had a self-serving agenda, and that the couple had better hire a doula, who would run interference for them if the team tried to talk them into something.

  This is not some kind of fantasy scenario—these patients exist, and I've cared for quite a few of them. Now, think about this for a minute. You've got two laypeople who've taken a four- to eight-week childbirth class and read a handful of books trying to make important decisions that they don't have the qualifications to make. Sound crazy? It is. Luckily, most of the time I've been able to gain their trust and explain the realities of their situation. After a while it began to sink in that I was not the enemy, that I was actually on their side and had the same objectives.

- **Listen to their advice.** Remember, the health care professionals at your hospital assist in delivering babies every day. They know when labor is progressing efficiently, and when you've hit a logjam. If they see that you're no longer coping and are suffering in labor, something needs to change. Nurses are particularly adept in helping you to move toward a new option for coping and/or pain management. They do take pride and find professional satisfaction in making a difference.
- **Don't be afraid to ask questions.** Ask the nurse's opinion on what she thinks would be the best move to make next. Back in the shower? Walk the halls? Medication/epidural? How about pushing and episiotomies? Even if that particular nurse ends up not being with you for that stage, she can still discuss it with you and then pass along your thoughts to your nurse on the next shift.
- **Be flexible.** Having an image of your ideal birth is fine, but remember that only the stork knows for sure how labor and delivery are going to go, so be prepared to change your plans along the way as necessary.
- **Learn to understand their language.** Throughout this chapter we covered a lot of terms and phrases the medical team may use. Having at least some idea what they're talking about can help you feel less like things are happening *to* you and give you the tools to communicate throughout the process.

MAKING A CHANGE

In the unlikely event that there's a chemical imbalance between your wife (or you) and your nurse, or if it's just not a good match for whatever reason, take a walk out to the nurses' station and ask to speak with the charge nurse. Explain the situation and *ask* for her help. I'm emphasizing "ask" because there's a big difference between asking and banging your fist on the countertop, demanding a change. The charge nurse will try her best to accommodate you. Keep in mind, though, that depending on the business of the shift and staffing levels, that could take some time. Although they want your experience to be a good one, remember, you're in a hospital, *not* a hotel. Your needs may not be their priority at that precise moment and you may have to be patient.

- **Make some introductions.** Each time a new member of the health care team (new shift = new nurse) comes into your room, remember to introduce yourselves. If you brought someone else in with you for added support (family, friend, or doula) introduce them as well.
- **Bring them up to speed.** Give them the short version of what some of your labor goals are. Tell them anything that will give them a better sense of you as individuals. For example, "Her sister had a baby last year and told us that she screamed bloody murder for two hours and that she will never give birth again," or "We had four miscarriages and can't believe we finally made it this far," or "My father is a physician, and he's been filling our heads with hospital war stories," or "I am very afraid of needles and although I want to be supportive, I don't know if I can or should be in the room if she needs a needle of any kind." If you ask, your nurse may be able to help you write your script, from getting you an epidural when the anesthesiologist has an opening, to respecting and supporting your desire to avoid interventions.

- **Get yourselves up to speed.** Your nurse knows what's going on outside the labor room and can fill you in on things like whether the shift is especially busy, the number of patients who are requesting epidurals, how many are going in for cesareans, and so on. The answers to these questions can have a big impact on the kind of care you get. For example, if it's a busy shift and everyone seems to be requesting epidurals, you may have a bit of a wait if you decide you want one too.
- **Speak up.** Your medical team will do their best on your behalf, but they're not mind readers. When your doctor whips into the room for a quick check and it's really important to you to know when he'll be back, ask! If Dad needs to go out for a few minutes, ask the nurse if she'll stay with you while he's gone.
- **Feed them.** If you're going down to the cafeteria or outside the hospital to get something to eat, offer to bring something back for your nurse. (If they say no, bring back a little something anyway. Nurses work long hours and often don't get a meal break.)
- **Show appreciation.** A simple "thank you" goes a long way. The more they feel that they're being treated with the respect they're due, the more motivated they'll be to go all out for you.
- **Be careful what you read.** There's a lot of pregnancy- and birth-related material out there that seems to exist for no other purpose than to scare the hell out of expectant parents. I know you're going to be reading other books, magazines, and Web pages, but carefully consider the source. There are a lot of self-proclaimed experts out there feeding misinformation to unsuspecting readers. These folks usually have good intentions, but their beliefs too often are not

grounded in experience or evidence. Unfortunately, the passion and conviction with which they write makes their opinions seem like fact.

- **Be careful what you listen to.** Well-intentioned friends, family, and even the strangers who weren't satisfied to just come up and rub your belly may want to tell you their childbirth stories. It seems to be human nature to want to share the nittiest and the grittiest last little detail. These people don't mean to increase your concern and anxiety, but they do. Demystify and clarify—get the real answers from the people who know. If you have *any* questions about *anything* you hear, talk to your OB or midwife. Health care professionals spend a lot of time doing what obstetrician Laurie Green calls damage control, listening to patients recount their most recent bit of monumentally wrong information and re-educating them with the facts. Your medical team's goal (and responsibility) is to make sure you have the most accurate information so that *together* you can make the best medical decisions for you and your baby.

CHAPTER 7

Having a Healthy Baby and *No* Regrets

WHAT YOU'LL LEARN IN THIS CHAPTER:

- Overcoming the myth of the perfect birth
- The secrets to having a no-regret birth experience
- Birth plans and why you don't need one
- Your first few days as parents. Okay, so *now* what do we do?

AS YOU KNOW by now, I believe that avoiding epidurals and medical interventions is an excellent goal—but only in the same way that climbing a very tall mountain is an excellent goal: For some people, it's great; for others it simply isn't doable. Or desirable. (Take me, for instance. I'm the feet-planted-firmly-on-the-ground type and I know my limitations. When it comes to rappelling or skydiving or bungee jumping, I'm not signing up, at least not in this lifetime. A nice, long, slow marathon is more my speed.)

I know the mountain-climbing analogy may seem a little far-fetched—after all, millions of women have babies every year, while most people don't climb anything higher than a few flights of stairs. But there are a lot of similarities, so let me give you some examples of the many ways that having a low- or no-intervention birth is (and should be) like climbing a mountain.

- Your ultimate goal is to have a safe experience and a memory you'll never forget, a feeling of pride and accomplishment that you'll treasure your whole life.
- You need to spend a lot of time preparing—physically and mentally—for the big event. You'll read books, take courses, and listen to the stories of people who've been there, gathering their advice and recommendations, and learning from their experiences.
- You need to have a well-trained, professional support team to guide you—people who've done it many, many times before and who know how to help. You need to know who each of these people is and what his or her role is. Most important, you'll need to trust that everyone on your team knows how to do his or her job and has your best interests at heart.
- You need to understand all your options, *and* you need to prepare a plan B (and C and D), just in case something unexpected comes up. You're confident that the experts will help you make the most responsible decisions every step of the way.
- You need to appreciate and take advantage of technological advances. Many high-elevation mountaineers, for instance, want the challenge of making low- or no-tech ascents. But if the need were to arise, none of them would turn up his nose at portable oxygen, warmer clothing, better climbing boots, or rescue helicopters—all of which have saved many lives. The same applies to childbirth. Try to do it on your own, but if need be, pain management and life-saving emergency procedures are available.
- You have an image in your mind of the way things will go, but you understand that there's not necessarily a direct correlation between the amount of preparation and the outcome. There's no question that having the right training and knowl-

edge, a good support team, and top-notch equipment can improve the odds of having the experience you want to have. However, they are not a guarantee. Once you're on your way—whether that's labor or the ascent itself—circumstances might come up that could throw a wrench into all those beautiful plans. (The difference, of course, is that with mountain climbing, if things don't go exactly as you thought they would, you can always turn around and go back to base camp. With a birth, you're having that baby one way or another.)

- Again, although training and preparation are great, the only way to truly appreciate the enormity of the physical and psychological challenge is to go through the actual experience yourself.

Unfortunately, the "natural or nothing" attitude we talked about in Chapter 1 refuses to die. As a result, instead of enjoying their new role as parents and basking in the sense of accomplishment that *they did it,* far too many couples are overwhelmed with feelings of disappointment and regret. For the next few pages, I'm going to explore some other sources of those negative feelings, and I'll give you some important tips that will help you avoid (or at least minimize) them. After that, I'll take you through your first hectic-but-important twenty-four to forty-eight hours as parents. Your physical and emotional recovery is going to be tough under the best of circumstances. Throw in a brand-new baby and a little sleep deprivation and you've got a breeding ground for feelings of failure.

Birth Plans

One of the dirty little secrets about labor and delivery is that things rarely work out exactly according to plan—especially with first babies. But that doesn't stop traditional childbirth prep instructors and many, many pregnancy book authors from recommending that expectant couples prepare a written birth plan, which they're supposed to take to the hospital and give to every doctor and nurse they see. I've assisted at over 5,000 births, and how any couple could possibly sit down a few weeks or months before their baby is born and write a detailed—and sometimes rigid—plan for the day of delivery is beyond me. A birth plan is in many ways a manifesto for your body, a list of demands that even the most motivated birth assistants can't guarantee will be met. Ask any labor and delivery nurse her response to being handed a formal, written birth plan. She'll tell you that it's a potential setup for having things go in the opposite direction. That, of course, leaves the couple shocked and disappointed. "After all," they might say, "we wrote down everything they told us to in class, and we practiced our breathing every day. What happened?" What happened was that reality set in.

> *I see it all the time—couples come in clutching their birth plan, unwilling to make any compromises. Then something unexpected happens that doesn't fit the plan (and that's almost always the case) and all of a sudden their entire experience is ruined. They argue with each other and with the nursing staff and the doctors, and sometimes even put their baby at risk by refusing a needed procedure because of something they read somewhere or heard about in a class. It turns what should be a positive event into something miserable for everyone concerned.*
>
> —BETTY Y., LABOR AND DELIVERY NURSE

Now let me be clear about this: I have absolutely no problem with having an *ideal birth scenario* in the back of your mind. In fact,

I think it's absolutely essential that you and your husband spend some serious time discussing how you'd like the big day to go, and imagining it in all its splendor. Have goals that allow for flexibility along the way. Just don't put them in writing. Unfortunately, for a lot of people, putting ideas down on paper is like carving them in stone—it's practically impossible to make any changes later on. And that creates two very big problems.

First, as we always say, only the stork knows for sure what the day(s) of labor will look like. If you're locked into one particular plan, you'll have a tough time reacting to anything that you haven't specifically covered. And even if your plan does address some potentially unexpected items, there's no guarantee that what you've got written down will be the best approach, given the wide array of possibilities labor can present.

Second, human beings tend to kick themselves hard when the "plan" fails. Especially female human beings. When things don't go the way they were "supposed to," it's easy to feel disappointed or that you've failed, that if you'd only done (or *they* had done) X or Y or Z, things would have been different and the plan would have been fulfilled.

There's a very fine line here. Nurses love it when couples come in with some knowledge and an understanding of the process—it shows they're truly interested and invested—and they love it when couples talk with them about their preferences and are interested in discussing options. Nurses are looking for *flexibility* from expectant couples. We know that unless you're an OB or a labor and delivery nurse, your knowledge is fairly limited—you can't possibly learn a decade's worth of practical information by taking a prenatal class (even one that lasted four to eight weeks) or reading a few books. And this is where the problems begin. Asking questions in an effort to understand your options is one thing. Trying to pull rank in the face of a true medical emergency or a situation you don't know anything about is another. It shuts down communication and diminishes the trust between you and the medical team. Worse still, it could put you or your baby at risk.

I have seen and heard about some of the most unreasonable things that have shown up in couples' birth plans. Here are a few of my favorites:

- **"Absolutely no cesarean."** If an emergency arises, sticking to this part of the plan could have disastrous consequences.
- **"No anesthesia, even if I beg for it."** What about for a necessary episiotomy or to repair a tear? I guarantee that these are not procedures you'd want to do without an anesthetic of some kind.
- **"No IV—I will drink plenty of fluids to stay hydrated."** Drinking fluids throughout labor is great. However, there often comes a point where either the mom or the baby needs more hydration than drinking can provide.
- **"No episiotomy under any circumstances. I won't need one, because we have been doing perineal massage throughout the pregnancy."** Believe me, if your doctor is at the foot of the bed and he sees that you're about to give birth to a linebacker, you're really, really going to *want* him to do something proactively to protect you and your perineum. It all comes down to hat size. And believe me, some tears are far worse than episiotomies, especially those that are either jagged or extend into the clitoris. As we discussed in the previous chapter, perineal massage is fine, but it simply *does not* affect whether you ultimately will need an episiotomy.
- **"My husband and I will be left alone throughout labor—the nurses can come in only when we ask them to—labor is a**

natural process and should not be disturbed." Do you think either of you is 100 percent qualified to assess how the baby is tolerating labor or whether you're experiencing any problems? Do you really want your husband to be doing pelvic exams? Seriously, though, if you're really committed to this, the health care team will work with you to accommodate your wishes as best they can.

- **"Newborn babies are pure and perfect beings. No medication will be given to our baby—no ointment in the eyes, no shots of vitamins, no testing of any kind."** Although babies are pure and perfect beings, they also require some specific care, often in the form of preventative treatment to keep them that way. I suggest that you talk with your pediatrician about these procedures. They may or may not be necessary in your case. As far as testing goes, the fact is that hospitals are required by law to perform certain tests and procedures on newborns (which ones depends on the state you live in). Not doing them could put your baby at serious risk. The March of Dimes (www.marchofdimes.com) recommends that newborns be screened for at least twenty-nine possible disorders. Talk to your OB, midwife, or pediatrician to find out which ones are mandatory and which others (if any) he or she recommends.

A Special Note about Cesareans

Cesareans are plan B, the *other* way babies are born. Don't get me wrong, I don't think women should get cesareans unless they're absolutely necessary. And if I were pregnant again, I'd work overtime to avoid one. On the other hand, if that was the only way I could get to the healthy-baby part, sign me up! It drives me crazy to hear that there are still childbirth instructors out there teaching expectant couples that a woman needs to spend time grieving if she has a cesarean. Grieving for what, exactly? The loss of her vaginal delivery? I can't think of a better way to get a new mom to feel let down, disappointed, bad about herself, as though she'd failed. And as a nurse, I'm convinced that there's a connection between those negative feelings and postpartum depression.

A BIT MORE ON DOULAS

In Chapter 3, you learned that your husband is the best doula you could ever find. In Chapter 6, we talked about how some doulas occasionally overstep their bounds and get between you and your doctor. As I've said, I've worked with many doulas (and know many more) who make valuable contributions to their clients. However, I think it's important that you understand how *some* doulas can contribute to the couple's feelings of disappointment.

The big problem is that some doulas have an agenda and believe that their role is to do whatever it takes to help the laboring mom deliver according to her birth plan. As a result, they tend to want to stick firmly to the original plan—long after the point where it's no longer in the mom-to-be's best interests to do so.

Again, in our view, your husband is your best doula. We advise our students to take the money they had budgeted for a doula and instead spend it on postpartum care (many people who provide this kind of care are, in fact, doulas). If you're still thinking about hiring a doula, please take a few minutes to review our guidelines for working with doulas on pages 131–133 in Chapter 6.

The McMoyler Method Solution: Prenatal *Conversations*

Instead of you and your husband getting locked into something by writing it down, I recommend that you have a series of in-depth *conversations* about the birth. Topics might include any (or all) of the following:

- Medicated versus unmedicated delivery?
- Epidural or try to avoid it?
- Will Dad be at the north or south end of the bed for the delivery?
- In case of a cesarean, does Dad stay with Mom in the operating room after the birth or go with the baby to the nursery?
- Will Dad spend the night in the hospital after the baby is born, or will he sleep at home? (If you're sharing a room with another new mom, this may not be an option at all.)
- If it's a boy, do we circumcise him or not?
- When labor starts, do we want to go to the hospital right away or will we try to stay home as long as possible?
- Hydrotherapy. Remember to get me into the water as often as possible—it really helped during the pregnancy.
- Don't forget to ask the nurse to track down a rocking chair.
- Be sure to call my parents, my sister, your parents, etc., with updates.
- Remind me that we can do this and that we have options.
- Please don't watch TV during labor; you'll get distracted.
- If I poop in the labor bed, don't tell me.
- Remember to ask our nurse to take a photo of all three of us after the baby is born.
- Remind my doctor that I really, really do not want an episiotomy, so please remember those warm compresses!
- Remember the breath mints. I'll go ballistic if you have bad breath.
- If I get really close to losing it, promise that you will get our nurse in there right away.
- Promise that you will stay with me, no matter what. Although if the baby has to go to the nursery, *go with the baby*.

- Remind me along the way how much I want this baby, and remember to tell me that we're going home with one.

I strongly recommend that you get yourself a small notebook (a paper one, not a computer) and jot down those important thoughts, ideas, desires, items to bring, questions to ask, things to remember, and so on. As your due date approaches, you can review the pages and act on them accordingly. Keep the notebook with you at all times—labor could start completely unexpectedly and you might not have time to run home and grab it.

When you've spent time talking together about the way you'd like the birth to go, discussing what's critical, you'll be far better equipped to articulate your goals and desires and share them with the health care team. Having ongoing conversations between yourselves and constant communication with the health care team also leaves your options open, keeps your expectations reasonable, and makes it possible for you to leave the hospital with what you went there to get: your baby. Nothing more, nothing less. No disappointment, no shoulda-woulda-coulda. Let me give you an example of the problems created by getting too attached to birth plans and the importance of remaining flexible.

I remember one couple who arrived at the hospital, birth plan in hand, and almost immediately announced to everyone within earshot that they weren't going to allow anyone to "do things to us that we don't want or believe in." Well, that certainly set the tone and put the entire nursing staff on edge from the get-go. Since they were my patients, I tried my best to support their intense need to avoid interventions through a very, very long labor. I persevered even when the mom-to-be lay exhausted, crumpled in a heap on the bed; even after sixteen hours of labor, when she wailed after I checked her cervix and told her that she was still only 3 centimeters dilated; even when her husband had the nerve to say to her, "Remember, you don't want to pump your body full of those toxic drugs."

We had all been through so much that I stayed over for another shift, just to see them through to delivery. I was there when her doctor came in to discuss the fact that labor was going nowhere fast and that she was putting her baby in jeopardy. I was there while we wheeled her bed to the operating room for her cesarean, tears of disappointment and frustration streaming down her face. Her husband looked angry and upset, and walked slowly behind the gurney, as if he were on his way to a funeral instead of the birth of their child. A short time later, a ten-pound, five-ounce baby was lifted into the world.

The next day, I went to visit them in postpartum. We talked for quite a while, and I tried to reassure them that they'd done their best with the labor and that the decision to have a cesarean birth was the safe and responsible one. Unfortunately, they were both practically in mourning. Instead of looking down at their beautiful baby, all they could see was that the birth didn't go according to plan.

Dealing with Disappointment

Of course, birth plans and the "anything but natural is failure" myth aren't the only contributors to women's feelings of birth-related disappointment and regret. Preconceived (so to speak) notions of the way things should be are also a big factor, in part because the phrase "the way things should be" can mean different—and sometimes contradictory—things to different people.

What may seem absolutely intolerable for one woman may be well within reach for someone else. And although it's easy to think that short labors and vaginal births are always desirable, while long labors, epidurals, and cesareans are not, life is rarely so black and white. For example, you might feel some disappointment if:

- You had a very long labor that ended in a cesarean.
- You were expecting a long labor but instead had a very short one, which went by so quickly that you felt as if you were in a car with no brakes, speeding out of control, with no time to catch your breath.
- You were planning to have a scheduled cesarean but went into labor early, and what was supposed to be an orderly, well-choreographed birth turned into anything but as you sped to the hospital, unnerved and off-balance.
- You wanted a no-intervention birth but found the pain too much to bear and asked for an epidural.
- You knew before you even went into labor that you wanted an epidural, but things progressed so quickly that before you knew it you were 10 centimeters dilated and it was time to push—too late for the epidural.
- Instead of going into labor spontaneously, you were induced.
- The doctor you saw for all your prenatal visits wasn't on call the day your baby was born.
- You avoided medication and interventions throughout labor, but your baby needed to be delivered by forceps or vacuum extraction.
- You wanted an unmedicated, vaginal birth and everything was going fine, but a sudden complication arose and you needed an emergency cesarean.

DadBox

If the birth didn't go exactly according to plan, your wife isn't the only one who could feel disappointed. There are a number of reasons, most of which have to do with the provider-protector thing that's so much a part of the way men are socialized in our society. First, no matter how much you've prepared, it's going to be hard for you to see the woman you love in severe pain—and to know that there's nothing you can do to make it go away. Of course, you understand that pain is part of the process, but deep down inside you may be kicking yourself for not having done more. Second, you may hold yourself responsible for any deviations from the ideal birth scenario. If you were planning an unmedicated childbirth and your wife needed an epidural or ended up having a cesarean, it's easy to feel that "If only I'd done A, B, or C I could have gotten her through it."

Feelings like these are perfectly normal, but it's important to get over them as quickly as possible. Time you spend second-guessing and criticizing yourself or focusing on your (perceived) shortcomings as a husband is time you can't spend getting to know your baby.

> *I was completely committed to a natural birth, but after more than twenty-five hours of labor I was only 3 centimeters dilated. I wanted to keep going, but I was too exhausted to go on. So I had an epidural and less than five hours later my baby was born. Now I go back and forth between being angry that I suffered through all those hours of contractions for nothing, and being disappointed in myself for being weak and giving up too soon.*
>
> —JESSA R., NEW MOM

Interestingly, older moms (including me) are especially vulnerable to these kinds of feelings. Many of the "perfect" birth scenarios that are bandied about by traditional childbirth educators are written for younger mothers, who typically have fewer complications and need fewer interventions. Too often, women who put off having children and whose bodies don't respond the same way younger women's do end up feeling that they've failed because they couldn't live up to some abstract standard.

Second-guessing yourself is perfectly natural—a lot of us are actually pretty good at it—and I wish there were an easy way to keep those negative feelings about birth from ever crossing your mind. Unfortunately, there isn't. There are, however, several approaches that can really help, either in the moment or sometime after the fact.

- Make the McMoyler Method slogan your mantra: "Healthy mom, healthy baby . . . however you get there." That, in a nutshell, is what it's all about. I've heard from literally hundreds of graduates who told me that repeating that mantra throughout labor made a huge difference in their attitude.
- Resist the urge to rewrite history. It's going to be very easy after the birth to look back and focus on everything that didn't go quite the way you imagined it would. If you do find yourself in this situation, I'm betting that if you take off your hindsight glasses for a minute you'll find that you made the best decisions and choices *based on the information that was available at the time.*

Putting It All Together: The Secret to a No-Regret Birth

I can't emphasize enough that delivering a baby is *not* a competition or a contest. Having worked with thousands of expectant couples, I know that if you follow the advice in this chapter, you'll have a very good shot at achieving what we promised in the title—healthy baby, no regrets. Because this is such a critical part of the whole experience, let me take a second to put all the pieces of the puzzle together.

- **Prepare for the birth.** You've taken a childbirth prep class and you've read this book. You know the terminology, and you have a good mental picture of the way you would like the birth to go.
- **Be flexible.** Even with all that preparation, you know there's no way to predict exactly what will happen once labor starts. So be open to the possibility that you may need to change course midstream, and feel confident that the people around you will help you make the best decisions for you, your baby, and your family.
- **Have prenatal conversations.** Talk about everything, anesthesia, cesarean, rooming in, pain coping strategies, overnight guests, laundry, and more. Have these conversations early and often.
- **Skip the birth plan.** The only plan you need is to talk with your medical team about your preferences. Resist the urge to write a dissertation.
- **Skip the doula.** Better to save the money and spend it on postpartum care at home.
- **Prepare for the postpartum roller coaster.** Too many couples underestimate the extent to which a new baby will turn their lives upside down and inside out. Being blindsided by new parenthood can aggravate—or create—feelings of self-doubt and inadequacy.
- **Allow plenty of time for your first postpartum visit with your OB/midwife.** In most cases, he or she will take you through

a blow-by-blow of the labor, explain why things happened as they did—anticipated and unanticipated—and answer all your questions. If you get overwhelmed at the hospital (which is extremely easy to do), that first visit can give you an invaluable feeling of closure.

Starting the Fourth Trimester: Beginning Your Adventure as New Parents

The Best Birth is designed to prepare you for labor and delivery. And because the first few weeks after the birth really are an extension of labor and delivery, we'll focus the rest of this chapter on you and your recovery. We'll start with what happens in the minutes, hours, and days immediately after your baby is born and before you leave the hospital. At the end of the chapter, we'll talk about how the recovery process continues when you get home. (We know you're going to have tons of questions about caring for your baby, which, unfortunately, we can't cover in this book. However, we've included a list of excellent resources on pages 245–246.)

Although there's definitely an emotional component to your recovery, it's going to take at least a few days for your feelings to sort themselves out after the high of the delivery and the thrill of meeting your baby for the first time. In the meantime, you're going to be preoccupied with your physical recovery. Unfortunately, many new moms are completely unprepared and have no idea what's involved. The sharp jolt of reality—that life may not return to normal for quite some time—can contribute to those feelings of regret we talked about earlier. So read the following sections carefully. Knowing what to expect will help you keep your expectations reasonable. More important, it will keep you firmly in the "no regrets" camp.

What to Expect after a Vaginal Birth

Immediately after you give birth, all sorts of things are going to be happening, many of them at the very same time.

Don't Forget about the Placenta

Your delivery isn't over until the placenta is out and the blood loss from this separation controlled. This will happen between five and fifteen minutes after the baby is born. Your OB/midwife will have the umbilical cord looped around a gloved hand and will give a little pull every few minutes to see whether the placenta has detached from the side wall of the uterus and is ready to be pushed out. (Most new moms completely forget that there's still one more thing to deliver and are surprised when they're asked to give one or two more big—mostly painless—pushes.)

Once the placenta has emerged, your OB/midwife will examine it carefully to confirm that *all* of it came out, because as long as any part of it remains inside, your body will think it's still pregnant and will continue to produce large amounts of blood. Left untreated, this could develop into a postpartum hemorrhage. If this occurs, the health care team will snap into action to ensure that your blood loss is minimal. Having a team of nurses pour into the room can be frightening, but rest assured that the labor and delivery staff have a lot of experience dealing with this kind of situation.

Once the placenta has been delivered, a new mom often will be given a shot of Pitocin, either in her IV or, if she doesn't have an IV, via intramuscular injection. This helps the uterus contract and can prevent unnecessary bleeding. If the placenta hasn't come out on its own within twenty minutes, the OB may need to manually remove it with a procedure called *dilatation and curettage* (D&C).

If you're interested, take a few moments to look over the placenta. It's fascinating (to some of us) to see where it was attached to the uterus and where the baby was inside the amniotic sac.

Immediate Postpartum

At this point, your OB or midwife can begin repairing any tears or the episiotomy (if you had either). If you have an epidural, they'll double check to make sure that you're numb enough. If not, you'll get an injection of lidocaine. Most moms are so fixated on their newborn that they aren't even aware that any of this is happening. In a couple hours, you may start feeling some cramping caused by your uterus contracting and/or perineal pain, which is the result of stretching, tearing, the episiotomy incision, swelling, or pulling on the stitches that are used to repair the cut or tear. Medications are available for the cramping; for perineal pain, the most effective remedy is ice. It numbs the area and reduces swelling.

Your nurse will do what's called *fundal massage,* which is a vigorous massage of your lower abdomen. Together with the Pitocin, fundal massage will help the uterus contract, constrict blood vessels, and reduce bleeding. While she's massaging, the nurse will pay attention to how much you're bleeding. Fundal massage will be done intermittently for the next hour or two, and the nurse may show you and your husband how to do it. If you didn't have one already, you'll get an automatic blood pressure cuff on your upper arm. If you had an epidural, that catheter will be removed within the first hour, and the Foley catheter that was used to drain your bladder will most likely come out at the same time.

The Feeding Frenzy Begins (Yours and Your Baby's)

You've lost a lot of fluids during the birth. If you had an IV before delivery, it will stay in, possibly until the next day. This will ensure that you get enough fluids, that your bleeding is under control, and that you don't need antibiotics or other medication. (Many women will have their IV removed as soon as two hours after the birth, but the decision to do this is made on a case-by-case basis.)

You will most likely be voracious. The nurses will bring you buckets of juice (and probably some snacks) to help rehydrate you and to give you the energy you're going to need to keep you from fainting when you get up and out of bed for the first time. The nurses will help you get the baby latched onto your breast for the first time. Anytime within the first hour is perfect, as babies are usually awake, alert, and interested. After a few hours, they go into a deep sleep and it will be harder to accomplish this introduction to breastfeeding.

During the first two or three days after delivery, you may have some uncomfortable contractions (often called *afterbirth pain)*—especially during breastfeeding. Ibuprofen will usually provide the relief you're looking for. But if you need something stronger, tell your nurse.

Your First Baby Steps

Do not get up without your nurse. She (and possibly your partner) will help you the first few times you get out of bed. If you didn't have an epidural, you can get up within an hour or so after the birth. If you *did* have an epidural, you'll probably need closer to two hours for your legs to completely wake up and be able to support you. When getting up, start by sitting on the edge of the bed, breathing deeply, until you get over any feelings of wooziness. Then slowly stand up beside the bed and stay there for a few moments.

At this point, don't be surprised if you have blood running down your legs, making a small puddle on the floor. This is happening because while you were sitting up in bed, the *lochia* (vaginal discharge caused by the shedding of the lining of the uterus) pools in the uterus. When you stand up, there's only one place for it to go—down and out. (During the first few days after delivery, lochia is like a heavy menstrual flow. It decreases each day, and over the course of a month, the color will gradually go from bright red to lighter red-pink to yellowish opaque.)

Your first trip to the bathroom can be quite an adventure. When you get to the toilet, sit down slowly. Don't be surprised if you are now passing clots, which can be as large as tangerines. This is uterine debris—your body is getting rid of everything it no longer needs, including all the extra blood that supported the pregnancy. Urine passing over the perineum can be quite painful—so much so that some women are afraid to pee after delivery—and the pain may make you hold your breath. Try not to. Instead, go back to the slow, focused breathing you did during labor. To avoid infection, change sanitary pads often, at least each time you empty your bladder. Rinse and clean your perineum with lukewarm water after every trip to the bathroom. Use a handheld shower, a squeeze bottle, or sitz bath. Wash from front to back, then pat dry with toilet tissue—no rubbing! Antiseptic spray or creams, or premoistened pads, may provide some additional relief. Now walk sloooowly back to bed and get some rest. You'll be doing it all over again in a few hours. Ice packs, which your nurse will be glad to bring to you, are heavenly on the perineum and really help reduce swelling in the first twenty-four hours.

You also need to poop. However, many women are afraid to bear down because they're sore and don't want to risk further pressure. That's exactly why you will be taking stool softeners before you leave the hospital (you'll also get some to take home). Not all women are able to accomplish the deed before being discharged. If you haven't gone by day four, call your OB/midwife.

Showers are usually fine as soon as you can walk after delivery—usually a couple hours. So are tub or sitz baths (this is where you bathe while sitting in a small amount of water; it can be done in a bathtub, or the hospital can provide you with a portable basin that fits on the toilet). Most women will have moved to their new room in the postpartum unit by this time.

Here's what you'll need to have at home: disposable underpads (ask your nurse if you can have a few to take home; if not, most pharmacies sell them), ice packs (frozen peas in a Ziploc bag work well), saddle-size sanitary napkins, one-size-fits-all stretchy disposable panties (again, ask your nurse for a few extras), plastic squirt bottle (which you'll get at the hospital), lots of clean cotton, washable, short nighties, and several pairs of athletic socks (this is not the time to wear new slippers—they tend to get mucked up).

WHAT'S GOING ON WITH YOUR BABY AFTER A VAGINAL BIRTH

- Immediately after the birth, your OB/midwife will clear the amniotic fluid from your baby's airway by suctioning his mouth and nose with a bulb syringe. This will allow him to take a nice, clear first full breath.
- The umbilical cord will be clamped in two places, and either the OB/midwife or your husband will cut it. If the OB or midwife made the first cut, Dad will still have the opportunity to cut the remaining segment over at the warming table; just let the medical staff know that's what you want to do.
- Your baby will be either lifted up onto your chest or handed off to the nurse (or possibly an anesthesiologist) to be dried off and assessed on a

warming table next to your bed. (This will depend on how you and the baby are doing, as well as how your OB/midwife generally does things.) Your baby will get an Apgar score (see pages 135–136 for a definition) and, if necessary, some oxygen to help get those lungs working on their own. (This usually means placing an oxygen mask near the baby's face for what's called *blow-by oxygen,* literally just a whiff.)

- Babies will get two security bracelets: one on a wrist, the other on an ankle. The bracelet will be imprinted with the mother's last name, the time of birth, the doctor's name, and an ID number. You and your husband will each get identical bands, which you'll need to keep on until all of you are discharged from the hospital. That's how the hospital staff can make sure you've got the right baby. Individual hospitals may have a variety of other security systems in place. You'll hear about them once you're admitted into Labor and Delivery.

What to Expect Immediately after a Cesarean Birth

Staying Ahead of the Pain

Immediately after the baby is born, you'll start receiving morphine sulfate through your epidural catheter. This will give you pretty good pain relief for the next eighteen to twenty-four hours and will allow you to breastfeed and usually stand at the side of the bed that evening. (If the morphine sulfate is not providing adequate pain relief, tell your nurse. She'll contact the anesthesiologist and get you some additional relief.) Some women have some itchiness or nausea as a result of the morphine sulfate (both of which can be counteracted with other medication, so ask your nurse). After the effects of the morphine sulfate have worn off, you'll receive pain medication on a regular basis. Take it—it's hard to chase pain! Following the schedule and recommended dosage will keep you covered with enough relief that you'll be able to feed your baby and be up and moving.

The hospital will have factored in that most women these days choose to breastfeed, so whichever pain reliever they give you will be compatible. The amount and frequency of the medication will decrease every day. During the first three days, before your milk has come in (there's a pre-milk, called *colostrum)*, very little of the medication passes through to the baby. When the baby is five or so days old, you'll be producing a lot more milk, which means more medication will pass through to the baby. However, by this time, you'll be taking significantly less medication than you were the first few days after surgery.

After your five-minute mini-bonding session with your baby, the surgeons will spend thirty to forty minutes sewing back together all those layers they cut through. Once the suturing is done, they'll most likely close the incision on the skin with tiny staples and apply a sterile dressing.

The nurse will do a vigorous *fundal massage* to your lower abdomen. This empties any clots and excess blood from your uterus. You'll get some extra-large sanitary pads, a clean gown, and a warm blanket for the ride over to the recovery room. (A team of people in the OR will help you move—very slowly—from the operating table to a gurney.)

You'll stay on the gurney in the recovery room, typically located on the same floor as Labor and Delivery and Postpartum, for the next two hours. The nurse will be right by your bedside—or at least nearby—the whole time. She'll monitor your blood pressure, pulse, bleeding, and response to the morphine sulfate. If your husband has gone with the baby to the nursery, he'll be able to come see you in the recovery room, give you updates on how the baby is doing, and then return to the nursery. The nursery staff will most likely bring your baby to you while you're in the recovery room. Once that happens, your nurse will help you get the baby latched onto your breast right there. If, for some reason, this doesn't happen, you'll start working on breastfeeding as soon as you get to your postpartum room.

Moving to Postpartum

When you're considered stable, you and your gurney will be moved to a postpartum room. You'll continue to receive IV fluids for the next day or two, until you can tolerate a soft-to-normal diet on your own. The Foley catheter will stay in your bladder for the next twelve to twenty-four hours (that's actually helpful—one less thing you have to get up for). Once you're in postpartum, the sooner you get up and move around, the better. But take it slowly. Expect some pain around the incision. Holding a pillow firmly over the incision while you get up will help you feel more secure. You'll also want to make a point of exhaling loudly when you stand up, sit down, or try to move in bed. We have a tendency to hold our breath or take small, shallow breaths when we're in pain. Loud exhaling will help decrease the internal pressure. Ask your husband to remind you to do this—it really helps. Keep your pillow over your incision whenever you move, whether it's to go to the toilet or simply to turn over in bed, as well as whenever you laugh, sneeze, or cough.

Pain and Hygiene

Even more uncomfortable than the incision itself are the gas pains that may develop after the surgery (some people say they're even worse than labor pain). With the manipulation of the bowels during surgery, *peristalsis,* or movement of gas through the intestines, slows down, which can cause discomfort. The best way to get peristalsis going again (and minimize gas pain) is to get out of bed and move around. Try walking the halls, rocking in a rocking chair with a pillow over your abdomen, or leaning over the bed while your husband rubs your back in a downward direction. Stay away from carbonated beverages and drinking from a straw—they'll only create more bubbles and will add to your discomfort. In most hospitals, you'll remain on clear liquids or a soft diet until you pass gas. (Don't be shy about reporting this to your nurse—once you have passed gas, you get to eat!) Your nurse will give you stool softeners. Take them. Pain medications can be constipating, and you can use all the help you can get in this department.

Coughing and deep breathing are an important post-op treatment. As with any abdominal surgery, it's going to be uncomfortable to take a deep breath for a while, so here's what to do: Place a pillow over your incision and hold it there firmly. Breathe in deeply, exhale, and then cough or clear your throat. This will expand the lungs and loosen any mucous that may have accumulated. Done regularly, this will help prevent any lung complications, such as pneumonia. (A reminder: Take as much medication as your doctor prescribes—you need to stay ahead of the pain. The more your pain is under control, the smoother your recovery will be and the easier it will be to breathe deeply, walk the halls, and feed your baby.)

Expect to have a vaginal discharge (*lochia*) after a cesarean birth. It will be bright red for the first few days, changing to a pinkish-brown and then to a yellowish color. You'll have to wear sanitary pads for a few weeks. Once you're home, if you have increased bright-red bleeding, pass clots, or notice a foul odor, call your physician.

DadBox

Helping Her after a Cesarean

Even though you're going to be the happiest new dad in the world, your wife will be recovering from major surgery. One of your major tasks is to make sure that she's as comfortable as possible. In addition:

- Keep in touch with the nurses—they'll let you know how your wife is doing and whether her recovery is on track.
- You'll probably be doing some running back and forth between the nursery and the recovery room. Be sure you take the time between trips to sit down next to your wife and fill her in on what's going on with the baby and when she's finally going to be able to hold him.
- Confirm with the nurse that she'll be available to assist your wife with breastfeeding when the time comes.
- When your baby does come to the recovery room, ask the nurse if it's okay to unswaddle him so Mom can see her child head to toe.
- Congratulate her on a job well done. Sometimes, with the blur of the OR and all the other activity, the fact that she just had a baby can get lost in the shuffle. Having a cesarean is no picnic, and she deserves plenty of accolades for having made the best out of a less-than-desirable situation.
- If for some reason the baby needs to stay in the nursery longer than Mom is in recovery, ask the nurse if she can wheel Mom to the nursery on the gurney. It's a fairly ambitious project, but well worth the trouble to get Mom to her baby sooner than later.
- If you were in a labor room prior to surgery, you (or someone you delegate) will need to retrieve your belongings from that room and bring them to your newly assigned postpartum room.

You'll be able to shower within a day or two after the surgery. Just don't spray water directly onto the incision (the first few times, the nurse will help you cover your incision so it doesn't get soaked). The *Steri-Strips* (industrial-strength tape) used to hold

DadBox

In the early days of new parenthood, you're going to spend a lot of time supporting and taking care of your wife and baby, which is exactly what you're supposed to be doing. But there's one important person who's often overlooked in all of this: you.

The fact that your transition to new parenthood isn't as physically demanding as your wife's does *not* mean that your life isn't changing at least as much as hers is. Becoming a dad will change everything. Your friendships will be different, and so will your relationship with your wife. Some new dads decide to rethink their work-life balance and change schedules or jobs. Others, who are worried about covering expenses, may suddenly get a second or third job. You might move to a neighborhood that has better schools, buy a car that has every possible air bag, sell your motorcycle, or even quit smoking. You'll feel a love like you've never felt before (loving a child is very different from loving your wife). You may feel jealous of the incredibly close relationship your wife and baby have, particularly if she's nursing and you have to go back to work. And you may feel completely incompetent as a father (if it makes you feel any better, your wife will probably feel the same way; babies have a way of doing that).

Too many men get so caught up in the idea that they need to be strong for their wife that they stifle their own feelings. But that doesn't make them go away. Instead, they build up and eventually come out as anger or resentment. The solution is communication. Remember those conversations you and your wife had throughout the pregnancy? Well, don't stop now. If you're feeling scared or overwhelmed or anything else, talk to her about it. She needs to know how you're feeling—whether it's good, bad, or indifferent—and you need her to know.

your incision closed should stay on for five to seven days. These help the scar to stay thin and well aligned but aren't essential to the healing. If they loosen up after a shower, pat them back on with your towel.

WHAT'S GOING ON WITH YOUR BABY AFTER A CESAREAN BIRTH

As we mentioned in Chapter 6, immediately after your baby is born, a nurse or pediatrician will take him to a warming table. If your husband wants to go there—to take pictures and possibly cut the remaining segment of umbilical cord—just let your nurse know. She'll guide him across the room so he doesn't get tangled up in the sterile field.

As soon as your baby has received Apgar scores, been dried off, had his airways cleared, gotten ID bracelets on one arm and ankle to match the ones you and your partner are wearing, and been swaddled, the nurse will bring him behind the drape to spend a few minutes with Mom (that's you!) and Dad. Your husband will resume his spot on the stool by your head and hold the baby for you to see and plant a few kisses on. This initial visit will probably last only about five minutes, but it's very important—a new mom really needs to see her baby before he gets taken to the nursery, where he'll stay for about an hour.

Life in the Postpartum Lane

Once all the excitement of the delivery—however it happened—is past, you'll be spending the next few days in a postpartum room (two for a vaginal birth, three or four for a cesarean). In both cases, the timer starts with the birth of the baby, not when you checked in. Most people will be in a private room, which includes a small bathroom and a pull-out bed of sorts for your husband to sleep on (although you should check with your insurance company; not all of them pay for private rooms).

Compared to labor and delivery rooms, with their comforters, armoires, curtains, and other homey touches, postpartum rooms are much smaller and plainer. (The logic, I guess, is that by the time to you get to postpartum you're focused much more on the baby, and your surroundings aren't nearly as important.) If you brought a blanket or quilt with you from home, now's the time to pull it out. It immediately personalizes your room and gives it a little more emotional warmth.

Your postpartum nurse may be working with a licensed vocational nurse and/or a nurse's aide. When they come in, introduce yourselves, just as you did when you were in Labor and Delivery. The postpartum staff will take good care of you, but don't make the mistake of thinking you're staying in a luxury hotel. They usually have a pretty big patient load—as many as four mother/baby couplets to care for—and they're very busy. Treat them respectfully and professionally and they'll bend over backward for you.

There will be a veritable parade of hospital staffers (not including your OB and your nurses) popping in and out of your room for one reason or another. There'll be the person with the birth certificate, hospital volunteers with goodies to buy, lactation specialists, a nursery nurse with paperwork to sign, your pediatrician to check in on the baby, a hearing specialist for the mandatory hearing test, a lab technician to draw blood, housekeepers to empty trash and bring fresh towels, the unit secretary with discharge papers, flower delivery people, someone from the cafeteria with a meal you ordered, and on and on. It's going to be a busy few days.

It's important that you empty your bladder frequently. A full bladder will affect the way your uterus contracts, the amount of bleeding you have, and your level of discomfort as time goes on. Unfortunately, many women, regardless of how they gave birth, have problems urinating. So here are some tips that will help you get those waters flowing:

- Try peeing while you're in the shower.
- While sitting on the toilet, put one hand under running warm water and, with the other, spray warm water from your "peri" bottle over your perineum.

- Ask the nurse to request some spirit of wintergreen or peppermint from the pharmacy, which she can put in a plastic container that fits inside the toilet bowl. The vapors waft up and can stimulate the urethra to relax.

DadBox

Your Role in the Postpartum Room

It may not be all that important to you that the room you'll be living in for the next several days be tidy and homey. It is to your wife. If at all possible, spend a few minutes before she gets there putting her toiletries into the bathroom, arranging her quilt and pillow on the bed, unpacking her glasses and cell phone, and so on. Then take a quick walk around the postpartum unit. Find out where the pantry and linen closets are. And ask about visiting hours. Will you need to make an appointment for the lactation specialist to stop by or is that automatic? Can local restaurants deliver food to your room? If not, can you bring it in yourself? If you're not familiar with the neighborhood, ask your nurse for some recommendations.

Keep the well-wishers under control. Right now you may think you're going to want everyone you know to stop by to see your new baby. Trust me, you won't. Of course, it's going to be hard to keep your immediate family away, and there will be a select group of people you'll want to invite. But you can always tell everyone else that your doctor advised you to get plenty of rest and limit the number of visitors.

Every time the nurse comes in the room to do *anything* with the baby, stop what you're doing and pay attention. Watch to see what she does, and then ask her if she'll watch you do the same thing. Take advantage of having a team of baby-care experts at your disposal. By the time you go home, you'll know how to change diapers filled with meconium (the dark green, sticky, hard-to-get-off-their-tiny-butts poop), what to do with the umbilical cord, how to take a temperature with a digital thermometer, how to get a T-shirt on and off, how to do a hospital-grade swaddle, how to use a bulb syringe to clean out your baby's nose or mouth. And let's not forget about holding, burping, soothing, handing off to Mom, and supporting the baby's head and neck. We say that moms have the baby and feed the baby; partners do *everything* else.

Don't get stuck in a situation where your only contact with your baby has to do with hygiene. In between some of the routine baby care tasks, make sure you get some quality one-on-one time with your baby—building the foundation of your relationship with each other. One excellent thing you can do almost anywhere is get some skin-to-skin contact. All you do is take your shirt off, put the baby (wearing only a diaper) high on your chest near your neck, turn her head to the side so she's looking out, cover her with a blanket, and prepare to melt. Your baby can now hear your heart beating, feel your chest rise and fall as you breathe, hear your voice resonating, and smell you. And don't forget to smell your baby! Take off her little hat and nuzzle. Babies smell amazing, like nothing else in the world.

Skin-to-skin contact is also good because it helps keep your baby warm. Newborns come from a controlled environment in the womb and are all of a sudden responsible for regulating their own temperature. By the time you go home, your baby will be pretty good at it, but for the first few days they can get chilly. Many a nurse (including me) has taken a baby with a low temperature out of the parents' room and down to the nursery to warm up under the heat lamps. You can probably avoid this, however, by having plenty of skin-to-skin contact. After all, you're the best warming unit around.

Earlier in the book we suggested that you tell people to send food instead of flowers. Unfortunately, not everyone will listen. The problem is that when all those arrangements get delivered to the hospital, you're going to be the one who has to figure out what to do with them when you leave. It's going to be hard enough trying to get your wife and baby into the car. Juggling seven crystal vases will just add to the confusion. So here's a solution: Leave the flowers behind. Give them to the nurses, the doctors, the housekeepers, and even to other couples.

Homeward Bound: Continuing Your Postpartum Recovery at Home

Conventional wisdom has it that postpartum recovery takes six weeks. In our experience that's rarely the case. Many women will continue healing—emotionally and physically—for as long as a year after their baby is born. Believe me, that comes as a surprise to a lot of women. Not being able to live up to your (often unrealistic) expectations makes it very easy for regret and failure to rear their ugly heads.

Your Emotional Recovery

Transitioning home with your new baby will be challenging. Prepare to move between feelings of immense joy and utter despair, exhilaration, and exhaustion. These mood swings are usually caused by a combination of the hormonal ping-pong match that's going on inside your body, a little sleep deprivation, fending off tons of unsolicited advice, and the normal challenges that come with feeding and caring for a newborn.

POSTPARTUM DEPRESSION

Most new mothers experience the baby blues—intermittent feelings of melancholy, crying for no apparent reason, and general moodiness. It can start while you're still in the hospital or anytime within the first few weeks after delivery. Baby blues are normal (though hardly enjoyable) and generally disappear on their own within a month.

About 10 percent of women experience more intense emotional symptoms, which are known as *postpartum depression.* Signs of postpartum depression can begin percolating inside a new mom within days, weeks, or even months after delivery. Symptoms may include:

- Inability to care for herself or her baby
- Crying spells
- Feelings of hopeless and/or despair
- Loss of appetite
- Inability to sleep or sleeping all the time

If you think you might be suffering from postpartum depression, contact your OB/midwife right away. Help is available. Treatment can include one or more of the following: hormone replacement therapy, counseling, antidepressant medication, and simply delegating a few of the thousand items on your new-mom to-do list.

Too many women don't get the help they need and deserve because they're feeling embarrassed or ashamed, afraid to let anyone know that they are *not* coping, that they feel like their life is over, that being a parent is harder than anyone ever said it would be, that they love the baby but don't know what to *do* with it.

A Day in the Life . . .

The first two weeks of parenthood are going to be pretty crazy. Here's a look at a typical day:

- eight hours breastfeeding: eight to ten sessions, forty-five minutes each
- three hours changing diapers: ten to twelve changes at about fifteen minutes each
- two hours trying to soothe your baby
- eight hours of constantly interrupted sleep
- three hours to do everything else (shop, clean, cook, shower, pay bills, etc.)

Trying to deal with all of that is going to be all-consuming. Here are some tips that can help you navigate the first few weeks—and keep those regrets far, far away. To help you remember, we're using the mnemonic NO REGRETS.

Network. Carefully choose the people who will support you in your new role. Try to do this *before* your baby is born so your team will be ready to snap into action as soon as you arrive home. With everything else that will be going on, the last thing you'll want to do (or have time for) is to make a bunch of phone calls asking for help.

Getting home is often a bit of a rude awakening—it's only then that you'll realize just how much was being done for you at the hospital. As a result, you may be surprised at how much you need and want extra help. We suggest that you and your husband focus on taking care of your baby. At the same time, surround yourselves with people who will take care of *you*. Let your support team help with shopping, cooking, cleaning, laundry, and so on.

Order baby announcements ahead of time.

- Request the envelopes before the baby is born so you can address and stamp them in advance. After the birth, all you have to do is phone the printer with the vital statistics.
- Have an e-mail blast ready to go ahead of time. Then all you need to do is fill in boy/girl, name, and weight, attach some photos or links, and click Send.

Run interference. Before you arrive home, put a detailed outgoing message on your voice mail that includes:

- Your baby's vital statistics: name, date and time of birth, sex, weight, length.
- Something to the effect of, "We're busy figuring out how to feed the baby and getting to know each other. Thanks for checking in. We'll get back to you as soon as we can."
- Consider setting up a Web site or a blog where you can post photos and announcements.

Enjoy the "first-week magic."

- Give yourselves some time to be alone with the newest member of your family. Enjoy as many of those moments as you can—you'll never be able to get those first weeks back.
- Take pictures and videos. Put on some music you love; stay in your bathrobe, sweats, and slippers; eat the gifts of food; and let yourselves fall madly in love with your new baby!

Gatekeep.

- Consider telling your friends and family that you can have no more than two visitors per day for the first two weeks. If they balk, you can always claim "doctor's orders!"
- Guests who do visit should bring gifts of food, not flowers! Believe me, flowers are pretty, but you'll appreciate a home-cooked meal or even a gift certificate for take-out even more. Don't worry that you might offend someone by asking for a specific kind of gift. The reality is that most people really do want to get you something practical—they just don't know what. So by coming right out and telling them what you need, you'll be doing them a favor.
- And no more of those cute baby outfits. There's no way your baby will ever be able to wear all the outfits you're going to get. If people really want to buy clothes, have them get something for a one- or two-year-old instead.

Respect each other. Dealing with a newborn is hard, hard work. The more you can help each other, and the more supportive you are, the better you'll be able to do the job. However, you need to understand that mothers and fathers parent in very different ways. Both are important, and neither is better or worse. Expecting your husband to do things the way you do them is a

DadBox

Welcome Home, Dad

When you finally bring your baby home, both of you are going to be like ducks out of water, going through some significant life adjustments. Understandably, her situation will be more intense than yours: Her hormones are bouncing around like ping-pong balls, she'll be getting less sleep than you, and she'll probably be responsible for the majority of the feedings. Her breasts are leaking, her bottom is sore, and your newborn child is crying. Throw in some financial pressures and the expectation that she'll be the perfect mother and wife, and it's no wonder that most women end up with the *baby blues*.

What all this adds up to is that you'll need to continue supporting her the way you did during the birth process. If she starts feeling that she's failing as a mom, it's essential that you remind her—often—that she's doing a great job. You'll have to bear with her short fuse as she adjusts to the demands of new motherhood. You'll have to make those calls for help—to the OB, the pediatrician, lactation consultant, housekeeper, and so on. You'll have to run interference, telling your parents (or hers) that they can't stay as long as they'd planned to—or perhaps asking them to come sooner. You'll also be in charge of crowd control, managing the well-wishers who are stacked up at your front door, the friends who've overstayed their welcome, and the constant barrage of unsolicited advice coming in from all sides. Here are a few more things you need to know:

- After leaving the hospital, discomfort from a vaginal birth is usually remedied with ibuprofen. A cesarean birth will require a regular regimen of carefully selected pain medication.
- Hemorrhoids can usually be treated with over-the-counter topical creams (Anusol and hydrocortisone). A severe case may require a prescription.
- Stool softeners are prescribed to all new mothers. Contact her physician if she doesn't get the "desired result" within three to five days of delivery.
- Remind her to do Kegels, which are an exercise done specifically to help strengthen the pelvic floor. The pubococcygeal muscle is the broad band of muscle that loses tone from the pressure of the pregnancy and birth of the baby. We recommend doing Kegels in a long, slow pace versus short and fast.

- Lochia is the vaginal discharge after both a vaginal or cesarean birth. Days one through three will be a heavy flow, days three through five moderate, becoming lighter over the next two to four weeks.
- To get a better idea of what her recovery is like, read the sections of this chapter on pages 204–209.
- Sex. Don't even think about it. I hate to be the one to break it to you, but even if she gets the green light at her six-week postpartum checkup, the last thing on her mind is having sex—and that situation could last quite a while. The good news is that although new parents have less sex, what they do have tends to be better than before. A few more important details: First, if your wife is breastfeeding, she could have some vaginal dryness for a while, so invest in some good lubricant. Second, foreplay has changed. The more you do around the house (baby care, cooking, dishwashing, laundry, and so on), the happier she'll be—and the closer you'll be to getting what you want.
- You can get the baby blues and postpartum depression too. And why not? You aren't sleeping, you probably aren't eating as well as you should or getting enough exercise, you're not having sex, and instead of *talking* about parenting, you actually have to do it. That's enough to get anyone down. In addition, new dads often experience a drop in testosterone—which is involved in regulating moods—right after the birth of their child (sounds crazy, but it's absolutely true).

The biggest difficulty with dads' postpartum depression is that it's very often overlooked. Dads are so focused on what's going on with Mom and Baby that they don't pay any attention to their own moods. If you're feeling melancholy, depressed, or not happy to be a dad, or are no longer interested in things that used to give you pleasure, do yourself a favor and talk to a therapist. Actually, you'll be doing your wife and baby a favor too: You can't be an effective caregiver if you can't take care of yourself.

great way to push him away. Encouraging him and letting him do it his own way will help him build the confidence he needs.

Educate yourself about child development. The more you know about what's "normal," the more reasonable your expectations for your baby—and yourselves.

Take five. Give each other time off so you can take a nap. Even fifteen to twenty minutes can make a huge difference between being sleep deprived and just plain tired.

Surrender. In our fast-paced society, expectant parents are accustomed to moving in one gear only—full speed ahead. With the arrival of your baby, you are now entering the "new parent zone."

This new chapter in your lives is all about transition. In order to transition smoothly, you must slow down. Parents need alone time with newborns. Even if it's just for an hour, that's the best way for you to learn to care for your baby in your own way.

Your Physical Recovery at Home

Much of the recovery process that started at the hospital will continue after you leave. There are, however, quite a few recovery-related things that you probably won't discover until you get home. Some of these will depend on the type of birth you had. Others are more general. Let's start with those. After that, we'll get into the specifics of your longer-term recovery from vaginal and cesarean births.

Every Mom's Recovery

- **Uterus.** Right after delivery, your uterus weighs more than two pounds. Over six weeks your uterus will shrink from the size of a watermelon back to its normal pear shape and size (a process called *involution*).
- **Bladder.** Some loss of control is common for the first weeks after delivery. Kegel exercises will help remedy this. (Doing a Kegel involves tightening the muscles you use to "hold it in" when you have to empty your bladder but there's no

restroom available.) Most women will pass large amounts of urine during the first few days after delivery. This is the body's way of getting rid of excess pregnancy fluid.

- **Bowel movements.** To encourage success, eat a diet high in whole grains and fresh fruits and vegetables. Drinking plenty of liquids will also help. Continue taking the stool softener—with a large glass of water—they gave you at the hospital.
- **Continued bleeding.** Once your lochia has subsided, any increase in bleeding following activity or exercise is a sign that you have overdone it. Have your desired brand of sanitary napkin already at home so your husband knows what brand to restock! (Tampons are *not* recommended.)
- **Nutrition.** Continue taking your prenatal vitamins. The average woman requires about 2,200 calories per day; add 500 more if you're breastfeeding.
- **Perspiring.** This is one of the body's annoying little ways of ridding itself of the extra fluid that built up during pregnancy. Sweating may be worse at night and may continue for several weeks.
- **Menstrual cycle.** Most women will resume their period between seven and nine weeks after giving birth, and egg production may return before the first menstrual period. Nursing mothers might not resume their menstrual cycle until they have finished breastfeeding, but keep in mind that breastfeeding is *not* a reliable method of birth control.
- **Weight loss.** The delivery of the baby, the placenta, and the amniotic fluid will result in an immediate loss of approximately twelve pounds. You'll lose another eight to ten pounds during the postpartum period, as your body returns

to normal. Once your physician gives you the go-ahead, resume a moderate exercise program to enhance continued weight loss. But be patient. It took nine months to gain your pregnancy weight, and it can take up to a year to get your pre-pregnancy body back.

- **Hair loss.** Anywhere from a few weeks to a few months after your delivery, it's perfectly normal to begin losing large amounts of hair. Eventually, your hair will return to its normal growth cycle, but it could take up to a year. There's no need to call your OB/midwife unless your eyebrows start falling out!
- **Non-breastfeeding moms (formula-fed babies).** You'll experience discomfort from engorgement (fullness caused by the milk) for several days, and you'll need to wear a supportive bra continuously. Ice packs help with discomfort and decrease milk production (a bag of frozen peas tucked into your bra works well). Acetaminophen can also help. Avoid letting warm water in the shower run over your breasts, as this acts as stimulation and will ultimately increase your discomfort.
- **Birth control.** When you are ready to resume sexual intercourse, you must use birth control. Again, breastfeeding is *not* protection against pregnancy.

Recovering at Home from a Vaginal Birth

- **Birth canal.** Sometimes the lining of the vagina is left with a "skid mark," or abrasion, from stretching as the baby passes through. This can cause a burning sensation while urinating and may take several weeks to heal. Breastfeeding moms will have vaginal dryness and some discomfort during intercourse for up to six months after delivery. This is due to decreased estrogen production during lactation. Think Astroglide!

- **Your perineum.** Grab a mirror and take a look. Most women are surprised to see that by the time they get home, most of the swelling is gone. Stitches, if you have them, are rarely visible (they're generally all on the inside and dissolve within ten days to three weeks). (You will occasionally see some black flecks from the stitches on the sanitary napkin. This is no cause for alarm.)
- **Hemorrhoids**. These can be troublesome! They eventually shrink, but until they do, you'll need some relief. Here are a couple of suggestions:
  - Ice packs can numb the area and help hemorrhoids recede.
  - Apply Anusol and/or hydrocortisone cream (available over the counter) topically.
  - For the "cauliflower patch"–style hemorrhoids, ask your physician about Cushing's ointment (prescription only).
- **Red flags.** If you notice any of the following symptoms after your vaginal birth, call your OB or midwife.
  - Foul-smelling vaginal discharge
  - Heavy bleeding that saturates one pad in an hour
  - Dizziness or lightheadedness
  - Passage of clots larger than a walnut
  - Fever over 100.3 degrees Fahrenheit (36 degrees Celsius)
  - Increasing uterine pain or severe cramping
  - Worsening pain in episiotomy or stitches
  - Persistent headache
  - Changes in your vision, such as spots in front of your eyes
  - Inability to urinate
  - Lack of bowel movement within the first week of delivery

- Area in the calf or legs that is tender, swollen, hot, hard, or red. This may indicate phlebitis or a blood clot
- Area in the breast that is hot, hard, red, and painful to the touch. This may indicate a breast infection
- Persistent baby blues/postpartum depression
- If you have any questions or concerns regarding your health

Recovering at Home from a Cesarean

Because cesarean birth is major abdominal surgery, the recovery period will take longer than with a vaginal birth. A typical hospital stay for a cesarean birth is three to five days. Recovery time at home is four to six weeks.

- **Caring for your incision and managing pain.** You may feel areas of numbness or tingling around your incision. It will take three to twelve months to completely heal. Take your pain medication on a regular basis so you're comfortable enough to care for yourself and your baby. When you can, switch from the prescription pain medication to ibuprofen.
- **Activity and exercise.** Generally speaking, try to get as much rest as possible. This will require additional support from your partner, family, and friends. For the first few days at home, don't do any more than you did in the hospital. Wait several weeks before climbing stairs, and hold off on driving until you're physically able to control a vehicle and are off of your pain medication. Don't do any heavy lifting for six weeks, and avoid vigorous exercise such as biking, aerobics, and running until you get the okay from your OB or midwife (which is usually six to eight weeks). Walking is the best

toning exercise to begin with. You'll need some additional help at home for the first few weeks. For some, this could be family and friends. Others will want to hire help. Spend a little time during the pregnancy researching your options.

- **Red flags.** Call your OB or midwife if you notice any of the following symptoms after your cesarean birth:
  - Fever over 100 degrees
  - Increasing lochia or saturation of more than one pad per hour
  - Redness, swelling, increasing pain, or discharge from your incision
  - Nausea and vomiting
  - Painful urination, burning, or urgency (sudden, strong urge to urinate)
  - Lack of bowel movement within the first week of delivery
  - Pain, swelling, or tenderness in legs
  - Chest pain or cough
  - Hot, tender, reddened area in your breast
  - Persistent or increasing perineal pain
  - Depression or inability to care for yourself or your baby

CHAPTER

8

A Stunning Childbirth Memory for Two

HAVING A BABY is the experience of a lifetime, and one of the cornerstones of McMoyler Method is to make sure that your memory of your baby's birth is indelibly positive. At the very least, you will leave the hospital feeling that you got *exactly* what you wanted. Unfortunately, research shows that at least one in three women actually has *negative* memories of her experience (given that about 4 million babies are born each year, that's a huge number of dissatisfied new parents). Those negative memories are largely due to feelings of failure, of not having had a "normal" birth, of having made a "wrong" decision somewhere along the line, and so on.

McMoyler Method grads are the glaring exception to this one-in-three rule. We get a lot of e-mail from our former students, and over and over, we hear that the birth of their child was one of the most amazing experiences of their lives and left them with a sense of pride and accomplishment. Of course, any experience that's filled with tension, pain, challenge, triumph, and joy can have that effect. This one, though, tops them all.

In this chapter, I'm going to share some of those stories with you so you can hear from real-life McMoyler Method grads—in their own words—about the birth of their child and how the experience affected their lives, as individuals and as a couple. (Some of the names have been changed to protect the family's privacy.) You'll hear from new parents whose birth story unfolded exactly as they imagined it would. And you'll hear from couples for whom *nothing* went according to plan. What they and everyone whose story falls somewhere in between have in common is that they left the hospital happy. Sure, they were tired, Mom's bottom was sore, or her cesarean incision was tender and the new baby was just figuring out how to exercise his lungs, but their overall feeling was one of joy. Another thing all these stories have in common is that they describe a shared experience—Mom is having the baby, and Dad is there with her, supporting and encouraging her and making critical decisions with her every step of the way.

A short disclaimer: Having become a mother twice myself, and having worked with thousands of expectant couples, I know that there is a wide range of birth experiences. As you read these stories, please keep in mind that the events they chronicle are unique to the couple involved and may or may not have anything in common with how your labor and delivery unfolds. It's also important to remember that not every OB or midwife has the same philosophy or does things the same way. So it's imperative that you rely on the advice of your OB or midwife for all questions about *anything* having to do with pregnancy, labor, or delivery.

We hope you'll find the stories you're about to read educational and inspirational. By internalizing the McMoyler Method message, you too can create stunning childbirth memories that will last a lifetime.

Pain

One might think that there would be a connection between the amount of pain a woman experiences in labor and her overall satisfaction with the event—that the more pain she has the less satisfied she'd be, and vice versa. Not so.

In this section you'll hear from three new moms who had three different approaches to coping with their pain—and three different experiences. Let's start with Marina (who bills herself and her husband, Kevin, as "the happiest parents around") and her description of giving birth to her baby, without any medication or intervention.

Marina, Kevin, and Baby Olivia

My contractions started off feeling like Braxton-Hicks (practice contractions) but the only difference was that I got a weird back sensation. I started feeling mine around 3:30 p.m. They were mild and pretty far apart in the beginning (thirty minutes). I was getting a manicure with my mom, no pain in sight! That morning, I also noticed the mucous plug; it made me nervous, but excited at the same time; finally something was starting to happen.

Since I was feeling like labor was starting, Kevin and I ended up going to dinner at my favorite pizza place (where contractions were pretty mild and coming every ten minutes or so). Also, I had two large slices of cheese pizza with garlic (which was a mistake because I had indigestion during strong contractions *and* Kev and I had *terrible* breath; I remember thinking about how awful it was during *really intense* contractions).

At 8 p.m. we headed to the hospital. We were supposed to be going in anyway for an induction, but I was actually, finally, in labor. The contractions were pretty steady, so they checked us in.

At 9:30 p.m., I was still only 1 to 2 centimeters dilated.

At 12:30 a.m., they checked me again and I was still 1 to 2 centimeters dilated. I was bumming because the contractions were coming pretty strongly at that point, and I was starting to question everything. Kev kept putting cold washcloths on my head and giving me drinks of juice between the contractions. The hospital had all this stuff, naturally! I was kneeling on the bed, which was nice because I was super tired and had a long night ahead. The doctor told me that most likely because it was a first pregnancy, I wouldn't deliver until the next afternoon—insane! The nurse turned out the lights and left us alone. She was going to check my cervix again at 4 a.m.

Turned out that wasn't necessary. Around 2 a.m., the contractions were really, really, really getting painful. They spread badly to my back and we brought a tennis ball to rub it, but that didn't work. Since the contractions were coming every two minutes or so, I tried to relax between them. This was *key* because I was actually able to get a few minutes of sleep in between. I wasn't thinking about an epidural at that point. But the contractions would be really strong in my back, which felt really, really awful—be ready for those. Kevin helped a lot by putting his whole hand on my lower back and pressing like crazy. That helped, but it still hurt.

Then around 2:30 a.m., they got really intense. Kev had to completely moan with me to get me through them. He had his face about two inches from my face and we would start with a *huge* deep breath, then these long moaning sounds. Every moan he did, I did. He saved me. Seriously, I would never have been able to get through it without him. Make sure your husband knows that he really, really, really is important in getting you through this. I laughed about this moaning response in birthing class but it is a very natural response to pain—highly recommend it when you are dilating at 10 centimeters. I would just do the sounds and try and push out as much breath as I could, which helped.

At around 3:30 a.m., when the contractions were insane, Kev and the nurse got me out of bed and I was going to try and do some positions around the room. I sat on the toilet for a while (good position), I leaned on a table for a while (good position), I sat in the rocking chair (*horrible* position, because I was so dilated at that point I could hardly control my body).

During one really huge contraction, my mom happened to walk in. The contraction monitor was reading 127 (the highest it reads) and it was not going any lower. This contraction seemed like it lasted forever with *no break*. I was obviously dilating to 10 at this point, but I really had no idea because last thing I knew, I was at 1 to 2 centimeters. I was wishing for an epidural but couldn't talk/ask/sit through getting it. I got through the pain because they seriously got me to remain really, really focused. My mom looked at the machine and said, "Hmmmm, should I go talk to the nurse? I don't think this monitor is working," and I'm like, "*Yes,* it is working." When the contractions come so strongly and don't give you a break, you should know that you are really close to the pushing stage. I almost started to panic on a few of them, but Kev reminded me to just follow his breathing and moaning. It felt like he was feeling the contractions also.

Kev and the nurse helped me get back in the bed, and I had another contraction, but with this one, something big slid out down there. Another nurse came in and everybody was in kind of serious panic mode (which I couldn't care less about because I was in such pain). I had pushed out the amniotic sac (which hadn't ruptured yet). They were very quickly throwing furniture out of the room (the rocking chair, the cot Kev was going to sleep on) getting ready for delivery.

I was moaning seriously at this point but Kev helped keep me calm. At this point, I knew I was going to be pushing the baby out soon, which seriously, once you know that, you can deal with any pain. My water broke and after that, I immediately started telling the nurses that I had to go poo. I didn't even care what I was saying, I just kept saying it. They said, "Marina, that's the baby coming." I was in hellish pain but knew I could do everything without drugs, etc., at this point. I definitely pooped on the bed (didn't care) and, no joke, once you feel like you have to take the biggest poop of your life, your baby is coming fast!

Kevin was telling me to "push, push, push," like he was a football coach, and the nurses were loud and coaching me through it too. One thing, most nurses are pretty hard-core and not sweet and friendly—I actually preferred them being like that because you don't want any small talk. You just want to push that freakin' baby out. They put an oxygen mask on me during the pushing, which was a gift from God. Definitely get one of those. I clenched my eyes closed and just pushed like a bowling ball was coming out of my ass for twenty minutes—it was insane! Then all of a sudden she was out—it was like pooping out an elephant.

I tore a little bit and they did stitches (numbed it first) but because I did it naturally, I was able to gauge how much to push without overdoing it (unlike those who have an epidural—they can't tell how much they're pushing or not pushing).

Some things to bring to the hospital for labor that really helped me: a handheld fan (I was *roasting* in the room—it felt like an oven), a sportsbottle with a straw for juice (you do not want to be drinking from a cup), an iPod with speakers (I listened to Jack Johnson for eight hours—definitely a good call), and glasses if you wear them.

Some advice:

1. I made sure Kevin knew that I wanted to know everything during the labor. When the amniotic sac came out, he was

good about telling me that the baby was okay, that her heart rate was great, etc. When the water broke, I asked about the meconium. You want to be informed.

2. Don't panic. Breathe and moan like you never thought you would. Some things work for you and some don't. Make sure to let your husband know that immediately.
3. Don't tell yourself that you cannot have the epidural because then you'll want it more and more. You never know how long your labor is going to be.
4. Really, really relax between contractions. Don't anticipate them, let them come and deal with them through breathing, etc.
5. Know all the lingo, because you'll hear the nurses using it and you'll know more of what's going on.
6. Once you have what feels like a ten-minute-long contraction that never ends, you know you're getting close to the end.
7. Don't worry about what anyone else thinks. When you walk into that hospital, all your ladylike manners are going to fly out the window—don't feel embarrassed about it!
8. Don't feel like the bed is your only place to be. Get up and walk around and lean on the tables and stuff. I think this was a *huge* turning point in my labor. The baby started coming because I got in that upright position—she kind of slid right down.
9. Giving birth, I think, is the most satisfying feeling of accomplishment you'll ever imagine. You will be so proud of yourself when it's done, no matter how you do it.

Like Marina and Kevin, Kate and her husband, Jamie, were also very committed to having a natural childbirth. Their story shows how important it is to stay flexible and focused on the ultimate goal.

Kate, Jamie, and Baby Kinley

It was really important to me to do my best to give birth naturally and without medication. I felt that I really wanted to experience this birth in all its glory and challenge. To cover every base, we had hired a doula; I spent months preparing my body for labor—lots of yoga, acupuncture, and trips to the chiropractor. I felt ready.

It is amazing when it finally happens. . . . Nine-plus months of planning and visualizing and preparing, and you still experience something that is way out of the realm of expectation. I had a birth plan and had experienced my labor in my mind a million times already. Evidently, I had a pretty typical labor and delivery, and yet I was still faced with feelings and thoughts and events that day that I had never been able to muster up in my head. . . .

I had my first contraction at about 11 a.m., while I was happily making my way through the farmers' market. It was three days before my due date. I remember stopping and realizing that what had just rippled through my body was not a typical tightening sensation like those I had had many times before. This one had a clear beginning and end, leaving me both excited and nervous. These very mild contractions happened about every thirty minutes or so for several hours. . . . I went about my day.

I met my husband for a long walk at about 4 p.m. At this point the contractions had moved up in frequency and strength. As we walked (it felt really good to be moving despite the contractions), we timed each contraction, noticing that they had become very regular, about every ten to fifteen minutes. We called my doula to let her know that the game was on, and we called our parents on the East Coast, who then booked flights to come out the next morning.

I knew that it was important for me to stay busy. We went out to dinner. We went to the store and got snacks and drinks for the hospital. We rented a movie.

By the time the movie was over (10 p.m.) I had moved from lying on the couch to sitting and rocking on the birthing ball, and being on all fours. This felt good. I remember realizing at this point that everything seemed exactly as I had imagined it. And I remember saying to my husband, "This isn't that bad!"

Soon after, we moved downstairs to the bedroom, where we dimmed the lights and put on the prepared "labor mix" CD that I had so creatively planned. I think we put on some reggae—I wanted this to be "*fun*" (hmmm . . .). At this point I was no longer just breathing through the contractions but was now letting out a sort of controlled moan, which felt good and helped me move through each contraction. I spent some time in the bathtub, which helped relax me a bit more.

At midnight our doula came over. From the beginning, her role was to support Jamie so that he could coach me. And although I wasn't communicating much at this point, I remember really appreciating that. Jamie was so present and relaxed and calm with me.

At about 2 a.m., I began to feel as though I needed to push, or so I thought. I got to the point where I knew I would feel more relaxed if I was at the hospital where the doctors were.

When we got to the hospital (after a challenging car ride in the back of our SUV on my hands and knees!) I was told that I was only 3 centimeters dilated—I could have sworn I was at 7 or 8! This was my first realization that maybe I had no idea what I was in for. . . . And I was disappointed, as I had really wanted to stay at home until I was close to pushing my baby out. I continued to breathe as we headed up to the labor room.

Once in the room, I went from the bed to the shower and back to the bed, for hours and hours. My music played. I had gotten myself into a rhythm at this point—breathing and moaning and coping. I remember Jamie telling me he was proud of me. I remember telling him that it was really hard.

Time is a strange thing when you are in labor. Nurses came in and out of the room to check the baby's heart rate. It could have been days or minutes. I had no idea.

It was really helpful during labor to have people talk me through the contractions. Jamie was right there with me, at times making the sounds with me and cheering me on. I longed for this each time a contraction came. It made me feel like I wasn't alone in this adventure.

I progressed to 7 centimeters relatively quickly. And then I seemed to stall. The doctor came in to check on me and said that she would need to break my water if I didn't progress soon. I didn't want this, as I was afraid it would make the contractions even stronger. Until this point, no one had asked me if I wanted the epidural, except for the nurse when we first checked in. I really appreciated this and felt like the nurses and doctor were supporting me in my decision to do it on my own. But I was getting tired and worn out.

I got to 9 centimeters slowly, or so it seemed. My water still had not broken. It was about noon.

Then it seemed as if I wouldn't open up any further. I was lying on my side at this point, and this was the only position that felt somewhat manageable. I thought I would want to be in the bath or on all fours or standing on my feet, but getting out of bed caused more discomfort and pain—the baby was really low and the pressure was unbearable.

This was the point in my labor where I had to give in . . . first to the moment (I actually fell asleep at one point, I think, or at least was in such a state of rhythm and coping that I went somewhere else physically and emotionally), then to the expectations (I remember saying to myself, "Okay, I've done this. I feel good about my efforts. I need help").

I was encouraged to work through several more contractions, which I did. And then I decided that it was time. At this point, I was afraid that when it came time to push, I would be too tired to do so. And I wanted more than anything to give birth vaginally, even more than giving birth unmedicated, so I asked for the epidural.

The nurse started me with a narcotic, with the hope that it would help me get to 10 centimeters and then I could push. But this seemed to do nothing to ease the pain.

After three hours at 9 centimeters I finally got the epidural. I was surprised that the doctor would allow this so late, but I think they saw how calm I had managed to remain and how committed I had been with my breath work. It was an easy epidural (and catheter), and like a light switch. Literally. I remember suddenly turning to my husband and doula and saying, "Wow . . . that was really crazy!"

The next hour or so was so remarkably different. I could feel and move my legs and could feel pressure when the contractions came, but I could talk and even laugh during them.

When I hit 10 centimeters, the energy in the room picked up again. Pushing was exciting—and actually not nearly as hard as I had imagined it would be. Each time a contraction came, I knew when to push because I felt the pressure, and so I still felt in charge of my experience. My husband and doula and doctor cheered (not my regular doctor, by the way). My water hadn't broken yet, and the first thing that came out with those pushes was the sack, like a water balloon, still intact. Finally it broke as I continued to push my baby through.

After an hour of pushing, our daughter, Kinley, was born! I was convinced that I was having a boy, and so this surprise was wonderful and emotional. She had meconium in her water, so the nurses took her first before she came to me. When she was handed to me, she latched on immediately. There is nothing to explain this experience. It is simply magical.

I tore slightly during her birth, and while I delivered the placenta and the doctor stitched, I stared. She was amazing.

I can honestly say that my birth experience was beyond my wildest expectations. It was amazing and wonderful, and challenging, and scary at times, and beautiful, and inspiring, and so, so, so empowering. I would even go so far as to say that it was fun (until the next time and I may retract that!). Yes, it was painful, but a kind of pain so unlike anything else. And while I did end up with the epidural, I feel content with my decision to get one, and lucky to have experienced both sides of the birth experience.

Nikki and Josh deliberately avoided making a firm commitment to a particular pain-management strategy. Nikki wanted to start off naturally but left the door open in case she changed her mind.

Nikki, Josh, and Baby Lukas

I was frying eggs the morning after my thirty-second birthday when my water broke. I had just showered and was wrapped in only a towel, hiding my enormous belly. When the dripping didn't stop, I put it all together. In a tone that was straining to hold back a dam of panic, I called Josh. In our state of excitement, even with all the preparations (lists written, bags packed, plans made) we still had no idea what we were doing. After much scurrying back and forth across the apartment, we finally managed to get dressed, gather our things, and get to the car. I can't imagine what would have happened if we hadn't prepared those lists.

Arriving at the hospital, we knew where to go (they had shown us on the tour a few weeks before). I checked in and saw a nurse. I began getting shaky with nervousness and anticipation.

Because I was GBS (Group Beta Strep) positive, I had to go to the hospital as soon as my water broke, so upon arrival I was not in active labor. Once I got a room, they began the Pitocin drip to get me to go into labor. (The nurses increased the Pitocin only a little at a time and it was nearly twenty-four hours later that I went into active labor!) During that time I had four different nurses and two doctors who worked with me—none of whom was my OB. One nurse asked me if I wanted to schedule an epidural for the next morning. I felt a little pushed to make this decision and told her no, I wanted to see how things went before committing to anything.

Although everyone was nice, it was definitely a hospital scene. I was in a tiny room and most of the nurses were very matter-of-fact.

Once labor kicked in (7 the next morning), I went from cheery to very serious in an instant. I felt like I was getting on a really scary roller coaster that I couldn't get off. I also felt like I had to go to the bathroom, and spent some time breathing on the toilet. I then moved to the rocking chair for a bit. Breathing and making noise was critical. It seemed like the natural thing to do. A deep "uhhhhh, uhhhhh" was what came out of my mouth. I remember staring at the ceiling lights, holding my husband's hands as I went through the waves. Josh was a bit stunned that it was finally happening, and it took him some time to figure out the best way to assist me and to focus on what was happening with me in the moment.

My initial plan with labor was to experience the pain for a bit and then decide at that point if I wanted to continue or get an epidural. After two hours I made my decision. A couple things pushed me over the edge: (1) A doctor came in to check on me and said that my contractions could possibly last until the evening (ten more hours—are you kidding?) and (2) our nurse mentioned that I wouldn't get any medals for having a natural birth and that if I wanted an epidural, I'd better tell her ASAP since the anesthesiologist was going into a cesarean shortly.

Before the epidural I was 2 centimeters dilated. After less than two hours of the early stages of labor and an epidural, I was 10 centimeters dilated. I was able to take a nap and then started pushing after the baby descended.

I was feeling much better after the epidural and was able to actually enjoy the birth, which was a nice surprise. I did shake quite a bit, like I was cold, and the epidural made me itchy. Fortunately, I was able to feel the contractions and could push along with them. I pushed for about an hour and then there he was, our son, Lukas. Since my husband could see I was pushing fine, he moved to the foot of the bed and ended up watching the delivery, which is something we did not plan. I also requested to have my new baby placed in my arms, on my chest, immediately after he was born, which was an absolutely unbelievable experience.

As I think back on that day, the healthy mom, healthy baby idea was always in my head, but I was never concerned that something could go wrong. Everything progressed naturally and when I finally went into active labor it all went pretty quickly. I always felt that I was in good hands with my husband present and the skilled nurses and doctors ready to assist me.

Thank Heaven for Dads in Labor

In Chapter 3, we talked about why Dad is such an important player. And Chapter 4 was written specifically for dads. Although most women have high praise for their husbands, the next two stories are among my favorites. In the first, Rebecca describes the wonderful feeling of discovering something new about her husband, David.

Rebecca, David, and Baby Amanda

The night that we went into labor it was a full moon, and let me tell you, when they say that it affects the internal rhythm of the body, they aren't kidding! There was a virtual population explosion going on that night at our hospital. Our nurse did her best to come in to check on us as often as she could, but, thank God, David knew what he was doing. I had no idea that he would be able to jump in to help me get through this the way that he did.

Trying to describe labor before it happens is like trying to imagine the taste of an amazing chocolate mousse before you have actually tasted it. Don't get me wrong, labor actually sucked—*nothing* like a great dessert—but I can now say (with labor a distant memory) that David was the frosting on my very challenging cake!

I thought for sure that I would be getting an epidural, but surprisingly, my labor was moving along pretty quickly for a first-timer. And I'll tell you what: It was the showers that saved me. David actually got in with me and was literally supporting me to stand up and slow dance with him. The other thing that surprised me was that I was willing to follow his cues to moan; those guttural sounds really do want to come up and out of your body. In class I thought, "Oh, right, there is no way that I could actually do that."

But let me tell you that when every contraction felt as if it was going to drag me through hot lava, I was willing to do anything to get to the other side. David really remembered that utilizing the rest in between the contractions is as important as coping with the pain of the contractions. He called the time in between the contractions the "safe side" and was really good at reminding me that I could let myself go in his arms and release my whole body. Anyway, we ended up pushing out a beautiful eight-pound baby girl, Amanda! We both sobbed as they handed her up for me to hold. Without question, it was the best day of my entire life!

The overwhelming majority of stories I hear come from new moms, which is why it's always so great to hear from a dad about how the birth of his child affected him. *So listen to Sam, as he describes helping his wife, Grace, bring their baby into the world.*

Sam, Grace, and Baby Cecilia

We have been meaning to write to you for some time to tell you all about the birth of our daughter, Cecilia. She was born on Tuesday, March 8, at 9:48 p.m. by cesarean section. She weighed in at a healthy seven pounds, five ounces, and measured twenty inches.

My wife had been diagnosed with pregnancy-induced hypertension, and I got a call at work from her on Monday, March 7, to tell me that she was experiencing one of the "danger signs" that her OB had warned her about: She was seeing flashes of light in front of her eyes. We were to get her to the hospital triage, where they wanted to monitor her blood pressure for a period of time. We were ultimately admitted to the hospital at 3 p.m. on Monday.

They hooked her up to an IV and began administering magnesium sulfate to prevent seizures. They first gave her a loading dose (amazing how quickly that was pushed through the IV) and then a lesser amount after that. Nasty stuff. At around 4:30, they gave her a drug to help ripen the cervix (it was well effaced, but still mostly closed). This procedure was repeated every four hours through the night.

On Tuesday morning at around 9:30, she was started on Pitocin to initiate contractions. Everything was going along just the way the process was described in your section on inducing labor, so we were very much at ease.

As Tuesday progressed, the amount of Pitocin was stepped up every twenty minutes or so, until we reached a point where my wife's contractions were coming too close together. They backed off the Pitocin a little to get the contractions back in line. At this point, she was still only 1 centimeter dilated. At one point later in the day, the doctor on call came in and tried to "snag the bag" to try to get labor progressing, but she was unsuccessful. By afternoon, we noticed a couple of dips in the baby's heart rate coinciding with my wife's contractions, and that got the attention of the staff. Our doctor paid a visit at around 5 p.m. and decided that she wanted to get a more accurate heart rate tracing. Out came the fetal scalp electrode (FSE), and it was successfully attached. This action had a twofold benefit: First, we had a hard-wired fetal heart rate, and second, attaching the FSE broke the bag of waters.

My wife began to feel the contractions much more strongly (probably due to the lack of the cushioning effect of the amniotic fluid), and the baby's activity levels decreased somewhat. Our doctor was on call that evening, and she began to grow concerned with how the baby was tolerating labor, and at about 8:15 p.m., the decision was made to deliver by cesarean. Needless to say, we were both a little nervous, and my wife was more than a little disappointed. I started reciting the mantra "Healthy mom, healthy baby

. . . however you get there." We had actually been saying that during the weeks leading up to labor, but we never expected to actually be in that situation.

As soon as they mentioned cesarean, our room was crawling with people: a couple nurses, our doctor, the anesthesiologist, and others were in and out. A lot of activity. My wife was given an epidural (a spinal was discussed, but it was determined to be too risky in light of her history), and it was amazing how quickly it was inserted. I was given scrubs and was told to put them on and wait in the hallway. I sat there and watched as my wife was wheeled into the OR. I guess I was out there for about ten minutes, but it felt like an eternity. I couldn't see a thing, as each time I exhaled through my mask, I steamed up my glasses.

Finally, I was escorted into the OR and was seated at the head of the operating table. I watched some of the operation over the curtain, and it was surreal. I was talking to my wife and looking at this yellow belly as if it wasn't even a part of her (really interesting to watch the operation). The next thing I know, the doctor pulls out our child, and I hear her first cry, and I get to inform my wife that we have a baby girl (we wanted to be surprised). I was absolutely beside myself with emotion, and I went over to the exam table (or whatever you call it) to help dry off our child, cut the remaining cord, and take a couple of quick photos.

We discussed several weeks before that if we delivered by cesarean, I would follow our child into the nursery while my wife was sutured and wheeled into Recovery. So I went into the nursery and stayed with our daughter. It was really special for me to spend time cleaning off our child and watch as she was bathed, weighed, and measured. I would highly recommend it to other fathers.

We were finally released to go home on Saturday morning, March 12, and we have been doing extremely well since.

Working with the Medical Team

Throughout this book we've stressed the need for trusting your doctors and nurses, and the importance of building good working relationships with them. In this section, you'll hear from two couples, both of whom checked into the hospital a little wary of the medical team.

In the first story, Renee, who wanted to deliver naturally, was worried that the hospital staff wouldn't support her and that the goals she and her husband, David, had spent so much time articulating would be ignored.

Renee, David, and Baby Elisheva

My husband and I decided very early in our pregnancy that we wanted to have an unmedicated childbirth, and we began looking around for information, methods, and classes that would help us achieve this goal. I read an obscene number of books that discussed every natural childbirth method under the sun: the Bradley method, HypnoBirthing, water-birthing, birthing with doulas, birthing with midwives, and so on. Many of the books I was reading were anti–medical establishment, and I became convinced that no one at the hospital would listen to me and allow me to have our baby according to my birth plan. By the end of my first trimester, my normally glass-half-full attitude had taken a turn for the worse.

Then the big day came and, boy, did reality set in once labor really got moving! I had a vaginal exam in the morning and was 2 centimeters dilated and 100 percent effaced. I was crampy for several hours after the appointment, and I realized that I was in labor around noon and I called my husband. I was extremely excited and could not believe that the big day was finally here. My husband, David, came home from work and we practiced some of our relaxation techniques from HypnoBirthing. We labored at home from noon until 9 p.m. This time was fairly easy and we were able to breathe through these early contractions.

We went to the hospital around 9 or 9:30 and my labor slowed slightly during the transition. I was 3 centimeters dilated when I arrived. The doctor wanted to send me home, but our wonderful triage nurse convinced the doctor that I should stay. She arranged a room with a Jacuzzi tub for our use during labor, and she called upstairs to determine which nurses were about to start the next shift so she could "reserve" a nurse who was really supportive of natural childbirth.

Approximately ten minutes later, as we were just beginning our journey from the maternity triage to the labor and delivery floor, I felt a sudden pressure and then a quick *pop!* as my water broke in the lobby of the triage unit. Within minutes, I had my first hard-core contraction and I knew that the game was officially on. David and I got to our labor and delivery room and I immediately got naked to get into the shower. My contractions were very intense and painful. I could not utilize any HypnoBirthing techniques. But I was able to find my voice and proceeded to scream at the top of my lungs for several hours. (It seemed like screaming to me; David kindly reassured me later that it was dramatic moaning . . . whatever it was, it helped.)

David was in the shower with me, pressing on my lower back and acting as a support for my heavy, tired body—he really kept me from completely losing it. Over the course of the next three and a half hours, I went from 3 centimeters to 10 centimeters. I spent about thirty minutes in the shower and then moved to the bed, where I labored on my knees, leaning heavily on a squat bar. David spent most of this time in the bed behind me, continuing to put pressure on my lower back, and feeding me ice chips in between my contractions.

Then I suddenly felt the urge to push. I was so excited because I thought that this final stage would be relatively quick and easy compared to the past three hours. I continued pushing on my knees for a very long time and quickly became overwhelmed and exhausted. I kept saying out loud, "I can't do this." What I meant was that I could not have my baby without medication, but I never vocalized this fear and I never asked for an epidural. David thought that I meant that I could not physically have this baby! He and our nurse kept cheering me on, saying things like "Yes, you can!" and "You *are* doing it!" They were incredible cheerleaders and never lost their positive attitudes. I was never once asked how much pain I was in and my nurse never suggested any sort of medication or other medical intervention. Once they could see the baby's head, I thought it would be any moment, but it ended up being another hour of pushing. My baby was stuck on the lip of my pelvis and was taking her sweet time coming out.

The doctor came in for the last forty-five minutes and he was amazing. His demeanor was calm and encouraging. He did not suggest the use of any intervention, such as an episiotomy, forceps, or a vacuum. He spent forty-five minutes patiently stretching my vaginal and perineal tissue with mineral oil. He finally offered me some lidocaine for the pain of crowning, which I at first turned down. A few moments later, he gently told me that the baby would not get any of the lidocaine, and I took the shot—and thank goodness!! It was so painful, even with the lidocaine.

Amazingly, after three hours of pushing, we welcomed Elisheva into this world without any drugs except for a lidocaine shot at the end—and only two stitches for a small tear. We felt incredibly supported by our hospital staff, and we felt empowered that we were given the opportunity to realize our birth preferences.

Our preparation and openness to making decisions to deliver a healthy baby ultimately enabled us to achieve our goals. We can't wait to do it all over again!

Unlike Renee and David, who wanted a natural birth, Courtney and Alex were much more in the category of "parking-lot epidural." Courtney wanted to get wired immediately but was concerned about the medical team's willingness to get her an epidural that quickly.

Courtney, Alex, and Baby James

When we were admitted to the hospital, my husband took the lead and right away made sure our nurse knew that I was *not* interested in having a natural childbirth, that, in fact, I was one of those who wanted the epidural ASAP. I was afraid she might judge me for that or think I was wimping out, but she was great. She contacted the anesthesiologist, who came in relatively quickly, and we got the ball rolling, so as the pain started to kick in, the process was already under way, and I was completely "hooked up to technology" by the time the heavy-duty contractions kicked in—which was exactly what I had hoped for. My husband helped the nurse when she came in to turn me over in the bed, and stayed really calm as we waited for the go-ahead to start pushing.

I pushed for two hours. Very tiring, and kind of strange because you can't feel that "urge" to push they talk about. I focused on what we'd talked about in class, which was "I'm constipated and want to move everything down and out!" (I remember in class feeling mortified that I might actually poop in the bed. I have no idea if that happened or not!) Our baby weighed seven pounds, eight ounces, and is quite possibly the most beautiful baby in the world!

Best-Laid Plans

If you've learned only one thing from this book, I hope it's that things rarely go according to plan. In Kat and John's case, the first of many unexpected events was going into labor more than a week early (a situation most pregnant women I know would envy).

Kat, John, and Baby Cameron

7:30 a.m.: Cameron's arrival was a bit earlier than planned (nine days), so needless to say, we weren't totally prepared. The battery-operated fan I'd ordered for the delivery room hadn't arrived (my big concern). John was out of town on January 31, the morning my water broke, or should I say *gushed.* After my usual morning pee, I got back into bed to watch *Today,* and that's when it happened. I wasn't sure exactly what was going on, but when it wouldn't stop I realized that this might be the start of it all. There was no pain whatsoever. I called John to tell him he'd better look into flights home ASAP.

8:30 a.m.: I called my doctor and explained what had happened. They weren't concerned. They told me to call back if I started having contractions or in twelve hours to give them status either way. I was supposed to meet a friend for coffee that day, so I called her and told her that instead we had to go to AAA to get our infant car seat installed!

10 a.m.: Lots of maxi pads later (fluid was still leaking, especially every time I stood up), we came back to my house and I decided to do a load of laundry and pack my bag for the hospital. Fortunately, my friend was able to stay with me all day until John got home.

1 p.m.: Still no pain or contractions, so my friend and I went to have lunch, followed by a trip to Walgreens to get more maxi pads

and trashy magazines (in prep for a long night). I also stocked up on small lollipops.

2:30 p.m.: Still nothing. Time to color my hair. (Decided I could at least look good in pictures at the hospital with the baby!) Thereafter, I just started cleaning and organizing, since I knew I wouldn't have any more free time for the rest of my life after the baby came. Couldn't believe that we actually might have a baby that day or the next . . . surreal thought. I was just hoping the baby would hold out until the next day, which happened to be my parents' anniversary.

5 p.m.: John arrived home (yea, relief). He put his hospital bag together, made himself dinner, and settled in to relax. I wasn't really hungry, so I had a few pieces of cheese and crackers. (I should've eaten more. . . .)

8 p.m.: Started watching *American Idol* . . . and the clock . . . tick-tock . . . till 8:30, when I called the doctor who was on call. He said to go to the hospital now, since twelve hours had passed and there was risk of infection. Since I wasn't having contractions, they wanted to start the induction process.

9 p.m.: We arrived at the hospital and checked in. This scenario was not at all how we'd envisioned it would be. In fact it was *the complete opposite* of how Sarah outlined the "you know it's time to go to the hospital when" scenario. I walked in on my own two feet, carrying my own bag, with no pain, and I could speak clearly.

10:30 p.m.: We got to our birthing room (huge, with a Jacuzzi tub). I was hooked up right away and they gave me a drug to start the contractions. I made sure that they knew then that the only thing on my "birth plan" was *epidural!* We settled in for a long night and waited for something to happen. John stretched out on the terribly uncomfortable cot and fell asleep while I read magazines until they came back to check on me.

2:30 a.m.: Nothing. I felt nothing. They gave me more of the contraction drug. I was *starving* now but of course couldn't eat anything. I also had a bit of diarrhea, which I think is normal during labor.

6:30 a.m.: Nothing. At this point they decided to give me something stronger (as we were now approaching twenty-four hours since my water had broken). I mentioned the epidural again, just to be on the safe side!

8 a.m.: John decided to go to Starbucks a few blocks away. On his way back he ran into a friend of mine who was at the hospital for a doctor appointment. She wanted to come up and say hello and since nothing was happening on the birth front, he invited her up for a quick visit.

8–8:30 a.m.: Needless to say, the contractions started while John was gone—out of nowhere. I breathed through two of them on my own . . . not too bad. No need to vocalize at this point.

8:30–10:30 a.m.: My friend came into the birthing room and proceeded to stay too long. I had to work through a few contractions while chatting with her and then finally had to tell her to leave! I found that standing and leaning over the side of the bed was a good position for me. John was then able to easily massage my back, which helped distract me. Contractions came on much more quickly at this point, lasting about a minute or so each, but were tolerable.

10:30 a.m.: I was already 5 centimeters dilated. The hospital staff was shocked at how quickly it happened. John was there helping me focus when contractions came on. Lots of moaning sounds . . . yee hawwww. . . . yee hawwww . . .

1 p.m.: I was already 10 centimeters dilated. Again, amazement by everyone that it happened so fast.

2 p.m.: I was ready to start pushing. I had pushed through a few contractions when it became evident that our baby was in distress.

The doctors were considering using suction but then concluded very quickly that they needed to get the baby out immediately. My doctor (who fortunately was the doctor on call that day!) said, "We're going to do a cesarean because that is the best thing for you and the baby. We'll have him out in two minutes." There was no more discussion about it—it's what we needed to do for healthy mom/healthy baby, so that was that.

Within seconds they pulled apart the birthing bed and rolled me down the hallway for surgery. The bed was bouncing off the walls—that's how fast they were moving me. It was really scary because we didn't know what the problem was but clearly it was serious. They threw some scrubs at John and said, "We'll be back for you in a minute." It all happened *so incredibly fast* that they were mid-incision when John arrived in the operating room.

2:54 p.m.: Literally two minutes later, our baby was born. The umbilical cord had been wrapped around his neck and shoulder. But he was fine. Looked and sounded good—scored a 9 on his Apgar test!

Needless to say, this wasn't quite the way we'd envisioned it all happening ("expect the unexpected"!). But not having an exhaustive birth plan certainly helped, as we really just followed directions. Since this was my first child, I didn't have the wisdom or experience myself, so we left it in their hands—they're the professionals and know best. (We felt confident knowing that our hospital delivers approximately 600 babies a month!) We also had the most outstanding nurse assigned to us. She was very knowledgeable, incredibly supportive, and really nice, so she really put us at ease. She explained everything as it was happening and would answer any questions we had. Fortunately, everything turned out just fine—we are very lucky and proud parents.

As wonderful as most medical professionals are, there are going to be some situations where the chemistry between mom-to-be and a nurse doesn't work out. In Arielle's case, having the wrong nurse got her whole labor experience off on the wrong foot. But once her husband, Jonah, was able to get another nurse, all the pieces fell into place.

Arielle, Jonah, and Baby Max

Although we got to the McMoyler Method goal of the healthy mom and baby, it was very different than I imagined it would be. First of all, we did not love our nurse, In fact, my husband needed to go out and request a different one. She wasn't dangerous or anything, but we just were not connecting. We had talked about this ahead of time, and my husband agreed that he would run interference for me. (I am a very in-charge kind of person, but everything we were learning was geared toward letting my body do its work, which means the mind must let go.) So I tried to keep that in mind as the contractions were picking up steam. My husband could tell that I was getting annoyed with the nurse. I can't quite put my finger on what it was, but when the nurse in charge assigned someone else, the whole picture felt more on track. My main message is that the hospital did seem to really have our best interests in mind. I ultimately got an epidural (what a blessing) and, with the help of a vacuum instrument, pushed an eight-pound, five-ounce baby out! Sore bottom and all, I would do it all over again!

Most couples—even those who have goals for an epidural—don't plan on a lot of medical interventions. Kristin was considered high-risk from day one, due to her high blood pressure, which is associated with a condition called preeclampsia. *For the last three months of the pregnancy, Kristin and her husband, Jeff, monitored her symptoms and reported her status to their doctor daily. As prepared as they were for interventions, they ended up with a lot more than they expected.*

Kristin, Jeff, and Baby Jake

Friday, November 3, one week before the due date of November 11: We went to dinner at PJ's Oysterbed, and during dinner and for several hours afterward, I started having contractions every fifteen minutes. None were too strong and after three hours, they disappeared. Drat, a false alarm.

Saturday, November 4: At 7 a.m., when I took my blood pressure, it was high. We called the doctor's office and they told us to come to Labor and Delivery right away. We were both pretty sure that this was going to be the day. We loaded up the car with our luggage and went to the hospital.

8:30 a.m.: I was admitted for lab work, urine testing, and NSTs (nonstress tests). One of our two doctors, Dr. Field, happened to be on shift for the day. What a wonderful surprise!

10:30 a.m.: The tests came back and Dr. Field said they were negative for preeclampsia—a slight indication of some blood issues, but good overall. However, due to the elevated blood pressure and the risk, his suggestion was to induce labor. We had an induction scheduled for a week later (November 11) anyway and the chances were very low (20 percent) that I would go into labor on my own anytime that week, as my cervix was not dilated yet.

After consideration, we decided to proceed with the induction, which would almost surely mean a delivery the following day.

Sunday, November 5: A good day to bring a life into the world! They explained the induction. First, they would start by inserting a drug called Cytotec into me four times over the course of the night to ripen, soften, and dilate the cervix. Then at 6 the next morning, they would administer Pitocin, which induces labor contractions.

1:30 p.m.: The doctor inserted the first quarter-pill of Cytotec. We were told that on rare occasions women may go into labor from just this cervix-softening pill. Well, I was one of those people.

5:30 p.m.: I was having regular contractions and they were getting stronger. However, my cervix remained closed.

6 p.m.: The doctors decided not to insert another pill, as the contractions were getting stronger and they hoped that would be enough to open the cervix. They continued to check in every few hours and I continued to proceed down the path of labor with stronger contractions. However, my cervix still would not open.

8 p.m.: Dr. Field and his team suggested that instead of starting the Pitocin at 6 a.m. the following day, we should start right then. Jeff and I deliberated privately on what we wanted to do. They told us that Pitocin increases the strength of the contractions dramatically as soon as it starts, and we knew we would be in for the long haul. We decided that to start right then would mean a night without sleep and to give birth in the night with no rest would be too hard. We *thought* (ha, ha) that the contractions were not bad enough and that I could sleep through them so I could be well-rested before the big 6 a.m. induction the next day.

9 p.m.: Oh boy! It was becoming clear that the contractions were too strong and we decided to set a time of 10:30 p.m. to decide if we would just go forward with the induction. We didn't want to waste the night by not sleeping and still having to go forward with the induction.

11 p.m.: It was *very* clear I couldn't sleep through the contractions, and we decided to move forward with induction.

Midnight: The doctors began administering Pitocin. It didn't take long before the contractions' strength and duration increased dramatically. The Pitocin adds a boost to what is already a painful process.

Monday, November 6, 12:30 a.m.: I was in severe pain. The contractions were only three minutes apart, lasting ninety seconds each. I was shaking uncontrollably and my body started evacuating everything.

I requested pain relief to take the edge off. They gave me a narcotic, but it did nothing to relieve the pain. I only felt woozy and disoriented, but still faced severe, finger-breaking pain as I clutched Jeff's hands and let out deep moans to move through the contractions. The narcotic was supposed to begin working within fifteen minutes, however by . . .

1:15 a.m. (forty-five minutes later), it was not having any effect and we needed another solution. One other solution was to use an epidural; however, that option was pushed back from the doctors, as they prefer to use an epidural only when the woman is at 3 centimeters or more, because an epidural can slow dilation. Jeff did his best to offer ways to reduce and distract me from the excruciating pain—calf and foot rubs seemed to work best. During the contractions I would close my eyes and Jeff would moan through the contractions with me until they subsided.

1:30 a.m.: Finally the doctors acquiesced and approved an epidural. However, they said, "Bad news: The anesthesiologist just went into a cesarean; it will be an hour." We said, "There has to be a solution." So they called the backup anesthesiologist, who happened to be a friend of ours. Based on our friendship she felt uncomfortable administering, so she decided to swap with the doctor in the cesarean, who turned out to be great.

2:15 a.m.: The epidural was finally administered.

2:45 a.m.: I started to experience pain relief. First it worked on the right side of my body and then slowly it relieved the left side.

3:30 a.m.: I was still experiencing contractions, but with virtually no pain. I *love* epidurals!

3:30 a.m.–7:30 a.m.: Magically both Jeff and I ended up falling in and out of sleep. Sweet relief!

7:30 a.m.: I woke up to a strange bursting sensation underneath me. I told Jeff, "I think my water just broke!" And it had. Unfortunately, I had lost my bowels as well. Jeff, being the sweetest, most supportive husband in the world, cleaned up the mess.

8 a.m.: The doctor came in to check the progress. Generally an epidural slows labor, so they weren't expecting much. However, much to their surprise and ours, in the past four hours I had dilated to 10 centimeters and Jake was in the +2 station. Wow! I was ready to start pushing.

8:15 a.m.: The nurse had prepped the room and called the doctor and said I could start pushing. Don't ask me how, but instinctively I knew to push from the lower abdomen. The nurse was so encouraging and said I was pushing extremely well. She couldn't believe how fast Jake was coming out. Then the doctor entered the room and could barely get his gloves on before Jake made his entrance into the world. Finally the doctor said, "Okay, a few more pushes." Jeff, who said he intended to only be near my face for support during the birth, suddenly got over whatever apprehension he had and was down between my legs saying, "Come on, honey, you can do it!" At one point the doctor said I could touch the head and I felt Jake's head as he was crowning. At this point, it was nothing like in the movies where women are screaming in pain. I felt so peaceful, so happy, and pain-free.

Finally he was almost ready to emerge. One more push and I felt the sensation of release, and Jake's head emerged from my body. Yet another push and the remainder of Jake's body emerged as well. The nurse asked if I would like him to be placed on my chest and of course I said yes. And there he was—this tiny hybrid of Jeff and me lying against my heart. He was crying, Jeff was crying, and I was crying. Welcome to the world, my beautiful, perfect baby boy!

Acknowledgments

Sarah McMoyler:

I was seventeen years old when I wanted to have a baby; the good news is that I was thirty four years old when I had my first baby . . . I thank my parents for their sage counsel in postponing that event and for going on to deliver four more children into the world. My passion for birth, babies and new families laid the groundwork for my career as a labor and delivery nurse, and I would like to express my gratitude to the hundreds of nurses, midwives and doctors throughout the Bay Area for sharing their knowledge with me.

It is my supportive husband Jeff, who, after being married for 25 years continues to champion all the ideas my overly active entrepreneurial mind generates, including the birth of a business. Growing McMoyler Method has been very much like raising a third child, and I could not have done it without him. My thanks to our eighteen year-old son, Luke, for being kind and caring, *and* running the San Diego Rock and Roll Marathon with me; it was just like the day he was born: exhausting and exhilarating! And bravo to our sixteen year-old son Corey for entertaining us with his music and Improv and for making us so proud, spending this year as an exchange student in Italy!

The women in my life have certainly played a role in this book being conceived and ultimately delivered. Berta Baumgardner, my thanks for your gentle, loyal friendship, and unconditional support. Gina Gabriell, so much appreciation for surrounding me with your art and living courageously. Daphne Blackmer, for arriving on my doorstep so many years ago to show support, and never stopping. Lori Sackett, our early morning runs have been a life saver; you are a constant source of inspiration. Mel McKee, my thanks for your rock solid friendship and helping to maintain a sense of perspective. Cathy Wills for sharing your gift of guided imagery; helping me to see more than meets the eye. Barb Silver, blessings for assisting our boys into the world and steadfast support ever since.

Charlene Stern, brand consultant extraordinaire, so much appreciation for your keen insight and vision and for helping set the stage for McMoyler Method in the twenty-first century. My compliments to co-author, Armin Brott, for his ability to take my life's work and develop it into beautiful chapters and also for introducing me to the Levine Greenberg Literary Agency. A special thank you goes to Stephanie Kip-Rostan, for instantly grasping McMoyler Method and helping the dream of a book become a reality. To our publisher, Da Capo Press, in particular, Renee Sedliar, whose guidance persisted throughout the editing process. Joan Nelson, my thanks for helping to keep the office spinning on its axis, even when the world felt a little shaky. Our attorney, Samuel Crump, appreciation for your lightning speed legal review of all matters book related.

On the medical level there are so many individuals who have been trusted, valued contributors to this process. On the obstetrical front, Dr. Laurie Green, my deep gratitude for reading every word of the manuscript, and providing feedback that incorporated your medical expertise with compassion. On the pediatric front, Dr. Brian Linde, for the heartfelt and integrity filled newborn updates. On the clinical front, Carol Kelly, CNS, for the investment of time to be sure we hadn't missed a beat. Our lactation consultant, Denise Barkasy, IBCLC for her tireless assistance to new families. On the psycho-social level, James Wright and Brett Beaver for providing a solid base to spring from, not only for those in McMoyler Method, but so many others.

Last and certainly not least, I am eternally grateful to the thousands of McMoyler Method graduates, for inspiring me, and for the opportunity to do what I truly love to do. Special appreciation to the families who so candidly shared their birth stories, further illuminating the miracle of birth.

Armin Brott:

Thanks to: Renee Caputo, Marnie Cochran, Kevin Hanover, Lindsey Lochner, Sarah McMoyler, Stephanie Kip Rostan, Renee Sedliar, Antoinette Smith, and Brent Wilcox.

Resources

Pregnancy and Childbirth

For Her

Curtis, Glade, and Judith Schuler. *Your Pregnancy Week by Week*

Iovine, Vicki. *The Girlfriends' Guide to Pregnancy: Or Everything Your Doctor Won't Tell You*

Odes, Rebecca, and Ceridwen Morris. *From the Hips: A Comprehensive, Open-Minded, Uncensored, Honest Guide to Pregnancy, Birth, and Becoming a Parent*

For Him

Brott, Armin. *The Expectant Father: Facts, Tips, and Advice for Dads-to-Be*

Simkin, Penny. *The Birth Partner*

Infant Care

For Her

Curtis, Glade, and Judith Schuler. *Your Baby's First Year, Week by Week*

Huggins, Kathleen. *The Nursing Mother's Companion*

Iovine, Vicki. *The Girlfriends' Guide to Surviving the First Year of Motherhood*

La Leche League International. *The Womanly Art of Breastfeeding*

For Him

Brott, Armin. *The New Father: A Dad's Guide to the First Year*

Brott, Armin. *Toolbox for New Dads* (DVD)

For Both of You

Cuthbertson, Joanne. *Helping Your Child Sleep through the Night*

Karp, Harvey. *The Happiest Baby on the Block*

Satter, Ellen. *Feeding Your Child with Love and Good Sense*

Sears, William. *The Baby Book*

Books on Birth-Related Controversy

Camann, William. *Easy Labor: Every Woman's Guide to Choosing Less Pain and More Joy during Childbirth*

Cassidy, Tina. *Birth: The Surprising History of How We Are Born*

Wagner, Marsden. *Born in the USA: How a Broken Maternity System Must Be Fixed to Put Women and Children First*

Wertz, Richard. *Lying-In: A History of Childbirth in America, Expanded Edition*

For further information and resources, please visit our Web sites.

- mcmoylermethod.com
- mrdad.com

Notes

2. Yes, Virginia, It's Going to Hurt

1. Wong, C., et al. 2005. "The Risk of Cesarean Delivery with Neuraxial Analgesia Given Early Versus Late in Labor." *New England Journal of Medicine* 352 (7): 655–65. Vahratian, A., J. Zhang, J. Hasling, et al. 2004. "The Effect of Early Epidural Versus Early Intravenous Analgesia Use on Labor Progression: A Natural Experiment." *American Journal of Obstetrics and Gynecology* 191:259–65. Segal, S., M. Su, and P. Gilbert. 2000. "The Effect of Rapid Change in Availability of Epidural Analgesia on the Cesarean Delivery Rate: A Meta-Analysis." *American Journal of Obstetrics and Gynecology* 183 (4): 974–78. Segal, S., R. Blatman, M. Doble, and S. Datta. 1999. "The Influence of the Obstetrician in the Relationship between Epidural Analgesia and Cesarean Section for Dystocia." *Anesthesiology* 91 (1): 90–6. All of the above cited in Camman, William. *Easy Labor: Every Woman's Guide to Choosing Less Pain and More Joy During Childbirth.* New York: Ballantine, 2006.

2. Camman, 81.Torvaldsen, S., et al. 2004. "Discontinuation of Epidural Analgesia Late in Labour for Reducing the Adverse Delivery Outcomes Associated with Epidural Analgesia." *The Cochrane Database of Systematic Reviews* 4 (CD004457).

3. Halpern, S. H., T. Levine, et al. 1999. "Effect of Labor Analgesia on Breastfeeding Success." *Birth* 26 (4): 275–76. Albani, A., et al. 1999. "The Effect on Breastfeeding Rate of Regional Anesthesia Technique for Cesarean and Vaginal Childbirth." *Minerva Anesthesiology* 6: 25–30. As cited in Camman.

3. Why Your Husband Is the Most Important Person in the Delivery Room (Other than You)

1. Diemer, G. 1997. "Expectant Fathers: Influence of Perinatal Education on Coping, Stress, and Spousal Relations." *Research in Nursing and Health* 20: 281–93.

2. Enkin, M. W., M. J. N. C. Kierse, M. Renfrew, and J. Neilson, with the editorial assistance of E. Enkin. 1995. *A Guide to Effective Care in Pregnancy and Childbirth.* Oxford: Oxford University Press.

3. Gibbins, J., and A. M. Thomson. 2001. "Women's Expectations and Experiences of Childbirth." *Midwifery* 17 (4): 302–13.

4. Tarkka, M. J., M. Paunonen, and P. Laippala. 2000. "Importance of the Midwife in the First-Time Mother's Experience of Childbirth." *Scandinavian Journal of Caring Science* 14: 184–90.

5. Palkovitz, R. 1985. "Fathers' Birth Attendance, Early Contact, and Extended Contact with Their Newborns: A Critical Review." *Child Development* 56: 392–406.

6. Moore, T., and M. Kotelchuck. 2004. "Predictors of Urban Fathers' Involvement in Their Child's Health Care." *Pediatrics* 113 (3): 574–80.

7. Mercer, R. T., K. Hackley, and A. Bostrom. 1984. "Relationship of the Birth Experience to Later Mothering Behaviors." *Journal of Nurse Midwifery* 30: 204–11.

Index